ALKALINE

DIETING

Understand Your pH Level with Easy and Delicious Recipes to Transform Your Health

DREW DORSEY

Disclaimer:

The information in this book is provided for educational and informational purposes only. It is not intended as a substitute for professional advice. Consult with a qualified professional before making any changes to your diet or lifestyle.

Table of Contents

Introduction to Alkaline Nutrition

What is an alkaline diet?

The alkaline diet is a dietary approach that promotes consuming foods believed to produce an alkaline environment in the body. While the concept has gained popularity, it's important to note that the scientific evidence supporting its benefits is still evolving.

The underlying principle of the alkaline diet is that by consuming more alkaline-forming foods and limiting acid-forming foods, you can help balance your body's pH level. Proponents of the diet often claim that an alkaline environment can improve overall health, boost energy, and reduce the risk of chronic diseases.

Benefits of an alkaline diet

While the scientific evidence for the benefits of the alkaline diet is mixed, many proponents claim that it can:

Improve digestion: By reducing acidity in the digestive system, the alkaline diet may alleviate symptoms like heartburn, acid reflux, and bloating.

Boost energy levels: Proponents suggest that an alkaline diet can enhance energy production by optimizing cellular function.

Support weight loss: Some believe that an alkaline diet can help with weight management by promoting metabolism and reducing inflammation.

Enhance skin health: By reducing acidity in the body, the alkaline diet may contribute to clearer, healthier skin.

Strengthen the immune system: A balanced pH level is believed to support a strong immune response, helping the body fight off infections and diseases.

It's important to note that while these benefits are often claimed, more rigorous scientific studies are needed to fully understand the extent to which an alkaline diet can impact these areas.

The acid-base balance in the body

The human body strives to maintain a delicate balance between acidic and alkaline substances. This balance, known as pH, is crucial for optimal bodily functions. A slightly alkaline pH is generally considered ideal for most bodily processes.

Acids are chemicals that emit hydrogen ions, whereas bases (alkaline substances) receive them. When the body's pH becomes too acidic, it can lead to various health issues. Conversely, an excessively alkaline environment can also be harmful.

The kidneys and lungs play significant roles in regulating the body's pH. They work together to remove excess acids and maintain a balanced environment.

Common misconceptions about the alkaline diet

Despite its popularity, the alkaline diet is surrounded by several misconceptions. Here are some common misunderstandings:

Strict adherence: The alkaline diet doesn't require strict adherence to a specific pH level. A balanced strategy that emphasizes alkaline-forming foods is typically suggested.

Quick fixes: The alkaline diet is not a quick fix for weight loss or health problems. It requires consistent effort and lifestyle changes for long-term benefits.

Miracle cure: The alkaline diet is not a cure-all for all health conditions. While it may offer benefits for some, it's essential to consult with a healthcare professional for personalized advice.

Oversimplification: The concept of acidity and alkalinity in the body is complex, and the alkaline diet may not fully capture the nuances of human physiology.

The Science Behind Alkalinity

Measuring pH Levels

The concentration of hydrogen ions in a solution is gauged by pH. There are 14 points on the logarithmic scale, with 7 representing neutrality. A solution is said to be acidic if its pH is less than 7, and alkaline if it is greater than 7.

pH may be measured using several techniques, including:

A piece of pH paper is dipped into the solution in this easy and affordable approach, and the color that results is compared to a chart.

pH meter: A pH meter is a more exact and accurate device that measures a solution's pH using electrodes.

Litmus paper: Another popular technique for determining pH is using litmus paper. In alkaline liquids, it turns blue, while in acidic solutions, it turns red.

It's important to note that measuring the pH of bodily fluids can be challenging. The pH of saliva, urine, and blood can vary depending on factors such as diet, exercise, and overall health.

Acid-Forming and Alkaline-Forming Foods

Foods can be classified as acid-forming or alkaline-forming based on their mineral content. While the body's pH is primarily regulated by the kidneys and lungs, the foods we consume can influence the overall acid-base balance.

Acid-forming foods generally contain higher levels of sulfur, phosphorus, and chlorine. Examples of acid-forming foods include:

- Meat
- Fish
- Dairy products
- Eggs
- Grains
- Legumes
- Alcohol
- Carbonated beverages

Alkaline-forming foods are typically rich in minerals such as calcium, magnesium, potassium, and sodium. Examples of alkaline-forming foods include:

- Fruits
- Vegetables
- Nuts
- Seeds
- Herbs
- Spices

It's important to note that the classification of foods as acid-forming or alkaline-forming can be complex and may vary depending on the specific food and its preparation. Additionally, the body's ability to process and metabolize foods can influence their overall effect on pH.

The Role of Minerals and Vitamins in Alkalinity

Certain minerals and vitamins play a crucial role in maintaining a balanced pH level in the body.

Alkaline minerals such as calcium, magnesium, potassium, and sodium help to neutralize acids and maintain an alkaline environment. These minerals are abundant in fruits, vegetables, nuts, and seeds.

Vitamins can also indirectly influence pH by supporting the body's metabolic processes. For example, vitamin C is involved in the production of collagen, a protein that helps regulate pH levels in the body.

While minerals and vitamins are essential for overall health, relying solely on supplements to achieve an alkaline balance may not be sufficient. It's important to focus on a balanced diet rich in whole, plant-based foods to ensure adequate intake of these nutrients.

Alkalinity and Health

The Connection Between Alkalinity and Disease

The relationship between alkalinity and disease is a complex topic with ongoing research. While some proponents of the alkaline diet claim that an alkaline environment can help prevent or treat various diseases, scientific evidence to support these claims is often limited.

Here's a breakdown of some of the potential connections that have been suggested:

- **Cancer:** Some studies have explored the link between acidity and cancer, suggesting that a more alkaline environment may inhibit tumor growth. To make a firm relationship, more research is necessary.
- **Chronic diseases:** Proponents of the alkaline diet often claim that it can help prevent or manage chronic diseases such as heart disease, diabetes, and arthritis. However, the scientific evidence for these claims is often inconclusive.
- **Autoimmune diseases:** Some believe that an alkaline diet may help reduce inflammation, which is associated with autoimmune diseases. To fully comprehend the precise mechanisms at play, further study is necessary.

It's important to note that while these potential connections exist, more rigorous scientific studies are needed to establish a definitive link between alkalinity and disease.

The Impact of Alkalinity on Weight Management

The alkaline diet has been promoted as a potential aid for weight management. Proponents of the diet often claim that by reducing acidity in the body, it can help:

- **Boost metabolism:** A more alkaline environment is believed to support optimal metabolic function, which can aid in weight loss.
- **Reduce inflammation:** Chronic inflammation has been linked to weight gain and difficulty losing weight. By reducing inflammation, an alkaline diet may help with weight management.

- **Improve digestion:** A healthy digestive system is essential for effective nutrient absorption and weight management. The alkaline diet may help improve digestion by reducing acidity.

However, more research is needed to fully understand the impact of the alkaline diet on weight management. While it may be a helpful tool for some, it's important to combine it with other healthy lifestyle factors such as regular exercise and a balanced diet.

Alkalinity and Skin Health

Skin health is influenced by a variety of factors, including genetics, lifestyle, and overall health. Some proponents of the alkaline diet believe that it can improve skin health by:

- **Reducing inflammation:** Chronic inflammation has been linked to skin conditions such as acne, eczema, and psoriasis. By reducing inflammation, an alkaline diet may help improve skin health.
- **Balancing pH:** The pH of the skin plays a crucial role in its health and appearance. An alkaline environment may help maintain a balanced pH level, promoting healthier skin.
- **Providing essential nutrients:** A diet rich in alkaline-forming foods provides essential nutrients that support skin health, such as vitamins and minerals.

While anecdotal evidence suggests that an alkaline diet may benefit skin health, more scientific research is needed to confirm these claims.

Creating an Alkaline Meal Plan

Understanding Your Dietary Needs

Before embarking on the alkaline diet, it's essential to understand your individual dietary needs. Factors such as age, gender, activity level, and overall health can influence your nutritional requirements.

Consider the following:

- *Caloric needs:* Calculate your daily caloric intake based on your weight, height, age, and activity level.
- *Macronutrient distribution:* Determine the ideal ratio of carbohydrates, proteins, and fats for your goals.
- *Specific dietary needs:* If you have any underlying health conditions or allergies, consult with a healthcare professional to tailor your diet accordingly.

Balancing Macronutrients

The macronutrients carbs, proteins, and fats are all part of a balanced diet. The optimal ratio of macronutrients can vary depending on individual needs and goals.

Carbohydrates: These provide the body with energy. Complex carbohydrates found in whole grains, fruits, and vegetables are generally preferred over refined carbohydrates.

Proteins: Building and mending tissues depend on proteins. Good sources of protein include lean meats, poultry, fish, eggs, legumes, and tofu.

Fats: Good fats are vital for good health. Examples of these are avocados, almonds, seeds, and olive oil. Avoid excessive intake of unhealthy fats.

Incorporating Alkaline-Forming Foods

The alkaline diet emphasizes the consumption of alkaline-forming foods. These foods are rich in minerals that help neutralize acids in the body.

Here are some examples of alkaline-forming foods:

- **Fruits:** Apples, bananas, berries, citrus fruits, grapes, melons, pears
- *Vegetables:* Asparagus, broccoli, cabbage, carrots, leafy greens, spinach, tomatoes
- *Nuts and seeds:* Almonds, cashews, walnuts, sunflower seeds, chia seeds, flaxseeds
- *Herbs and spices:* Garlic, ginger, turmeric, parsley, cilantro
- *Legumes:* Lentils, chickpeas, beans

<u>To incorporate alkaline-forming foods into your diet:</u>

- *Focus on whole, plant-based foods:* These are generally more alkaline-forming than processed foods.
- *Consume a range of veggies and fruits.* Five servings or more should be consumed each day.
- Include legumes and whole grains: These are excellent sources of protein and fiber.
- *Limit animal protein:* While not all animal proteins are acidic, consuming excessive amounts can contribute to acidity.
- *Remain hydrated:* A pH-balanced body depends on frequent consumption of water.

Remember, the alkaline diet is not about strictly avoiding acidic foods. Rather, it's about finding a balance between alkaline-forming and acid-forming foods to support optimal health.

Shopping List Essentials

Must-Have Alkaline Foods

- *Fruits:* Apples, bananas, berries (blueberries, strawberries, raspberries), citrus fruits (lemons, limes, oranges), grapes, melons, pears
- *Vegetables:* Asparagus, broccoli, cabbage, carrots, leafy greens (spinach, kale, romaine lettuce), tomatoes, zucchini
- *Nuts and seeds:* Almonds, cashews, walnuts, sunflower seeds, chia seeds, flaxseeds

- *Herbs and spices:* Garlic, ginger, turmeric, parsley, cilantro
- *Legumes:* Lentils, chickpeas, beans
- *Seaweed:* A rich source of minerals and nutrients

Avoiding Acidic Foods

While it's not necessary to eliminate acidic foods, it's helpful to be mindful of their consumption. Some common acidic foods include:

- *Meat:* Beef, pork, chicken, fish
- *Dairy products:* Milk, cheese, yogurt
- *Eggs*
- *Grains:* Wheat, rice, bread
- *Legumes (in moderation)*
- *Alcohol*
- *Carbonated beverages*
- *Processed foods*

Tips for Reading Food Labels

- *When shopping, pay attention to food labels to identify acidic ingredients. Look for:*
- *Added sugars:* These can contribute to acidity.
- *Artificial sweeteners:* Some artificial sweeteners may have acidic properties.
- *Preservatives:* Certain preservatives can be acidic.
- *Processed ingredients:* Processed foods often contain acidic additives.
- *Acidic ingredients:* Look for ingredients like vinegar, citric acid, phosphoric acid, and lactic acid.

By making informed choices and incorporating more alkaline-forming foods into your diet, you can help maintain a balanced pH level and support your overall health.

Meal Preparation Tips

Easy Alkaline Recipes

Smoothies: Blend fruits, vegetables, and a plant-based protein powder for a quick and nutritious breakfast or snack.

Salads: Create colorful and flavorful salads with a variety of leafy greens, vegetables, and a light dressing.

Stir-fries: Sauté vegetables with lean protein and a flavorful sauce for a quick and easy meal.

Soups and stews: Prepare hearty soups and stews using alkaline-forming vegetables and lean protein.

Whole grain bowls: Build your own bowls with whole grains, vegetables, and a protein source.

Overnight oats: Prepare oats with plant-based milk, fruits, and nuts for a convenient breakfast option.

Meal Planning Strategies

- ***Plan:*** Set aside some time every week to organize your snacks and meals.
- ***Make a grocery list:*** Ensure you have all the necessary ingredients on hand.
- ***Prepare meals in advance:*** Cook a large batch of food on the weekend to enjoy throughout the week.
- ***Pack lunches:*** Bring your own lunch to work or school to avoid unhealthy options.
- ***Snack smart:*** Keep healthy snacks on hand, such as fruits, vegetables, nuts, or seeds.

A Guide to Alkaline Dietary Dining Out

- ***Choose wisely:*** opt for restaurants that offer healthy options, such as those specializing in vegetarian or vegan cuisine.
- ***Make inquiries:*** Ask questions concerning ingredients and cooking techniques without holding back.
- ***Order wisely:*** Choose dishes with plenty of vegetables and lean protein.
- **Avoid processed foods:** Be mindful of hidden additives and preservatives.
- ***Make substitutions: If*** possible, request substitutions to make your meal more alkaline-friendly.

Smoothies

Green Goddess Smoothie

Yield: 2 servings Prep Time: 5 minutes Cook Time: N/A

Ingredients:

- 1 cup spinach
- 1 avocado
- 1/2 cup Greek yogurt
- 1/4 cup water
- 1 tablespoon lemon juice
- 1/4 cup cucumber, diced
- 1/4 cup fresh parsley
- 1/4 cup fresh dill

Instructions:

- Blend all ingredients together in a blender until smooth.
- Pour into glasses and serve immediately.

Nutritional Information (per serving):

- Calories: 250
- Protein: 10g
- Fat: 15g
- Carbohydrates: 20g

Storage and Reheating:

- Remaining food can be kept in the refrigerator for up to two days if it is sealed tightly.
- Blend till smooth with a splash of water to warm.

Berry Blast Smoothie

Yield: 2 servings Prep Time: 5 minutes Cook Time: N/A

Ingredients:

- 1 cup mixed berries (strawberries, raspberries, blueberries)
- 1 banana
- 1/2 cup Greek yogurt
- 1/4 cup almond milk
- 1 tablespoon honey (optional)

Instructions:

- Blend all ingredients together in a blender until smooth.
- Pour into glasses and serve immediately.

Nutritional Information (per serving):

- Calories: 200
- Protein: 8g

- Fat: 5g
- Carbohydrates: 30g

Storage and Reheating:

- Remaining food can be kept in the refrigerator for up to two days if it is sealed tightly.
- Blend till smooth with a splash of water to warm.

Avocado Almond Smoothie

Yield: 2 servings **Prep Time:** 5 minutes **Cook Time:** N/A

Ingredients:

- 1 avocado
- 1/2 cup almond milk
- 1/4 cup Greek yogurt
- 1 tablespoon honey (optional)
- 1/4 teaspoon vanilla extract

Instructions:

- Blend all ingredients together in a blender until smooth.
- Pour into glasses and serve immediately.

Nutritional Information (per serving):

- Calories: 250
- Protein: 10g
- Fat: 15g
- Carbohydrates: 20g

Storage and Reheating:

- Remaining food can be kept in the refrigerator for up to two days if it is sealed tightly.
- Blend till smooth with a splash of water to warm.

Tropical Paradise Smoothie

Yield: 2 servings **Prep Time:** 5 minutes **Cook Time:** N/A

Ingredients:

- 1 cup frozen mango chunks
- 1 cup frozen pineapple chunks
- 1 cup coconut milk
- 1/4 cup Greek yogurt
- 1 tablespoon honey (optional)

Instructions:

- Blend all ingredients together in a blender until smooth.

- Pour into glasses and serve immediately.

Nutritional Information (per serving):

- Calories: 250
- Protein: 8g
- Fat: 12g
- Carbohydrates: 30g

Storage and Reheating:

- Remaining food can be kept in the refrigerator for up to two days if it is sealed tightly.
- Blend till smooth with a splash of water to warm.

Spinach and Cucumber Smoothie

Yield: 2 servings **Prep Time:** 5 minutes **Cook Time:** N/A

Ingredients:

- 1 cup spinach
- 1 cucumber, diced
- 1/2 cup Greek yogurt
- 1/4 cup water
- 1 tablespoon lemon juice
- 1/4 teaspoon salt

Instructions:

- Blend all ingredients together in a blender until smooth.
- Pour into glasses and serve immediately.

Nutritional Information (per serving):

- Calories: 150
- Protein: 10g
- Fat: 5g
- Carbohydrates: 15g

Storage and Reheating:

- Remaining food can be kept in the refrigerator for up to two days if it is sealed tightly.
- Blend till smooth with a splash of water to warm.

Oatmeal Variations

Almond Butter and Berry Oatmeal

Yield: 1 serving **Prep Time:** 5 minutes **Cook Time:** 5 minutes

Ingredients:

- 1/4 cup rolled oats
- 1/2 cup almond milk
- 1/4 cup mixed berries (blueberries, strawberries, raspberries)
- 1 tablespoon almond butter
- 1 teaspoon maple syrup
- Pinch of cinnamon

Instructions:

- Almond milk and oats should be combined in a small pot. Heat to a simmer on a medium setting.
- Cook for 3-5 minutes, stirring occasionally, until oats are softened.
- Stir in berries, almond butter, maple syrup, and cinnamon.
- Serve immediately.

Nutritional Information:

- Calories: approximately 300
- Protein: 10 grams
- Carbohydrates: 40 grams
- Fat: 15 grams

Storage and Reheating:

- Remaining food can be kept in the refrigerator for up to three days if it is sealed tightly.
- Use a microwave or stovetop to reheat until well heated.

Chia Seed and Coconut Oatmeal

Yield: 1 serving **Prep Time:** 5 minutes **Cook Time:** 5 minutes

Ingredients:

- 1/4 cup rolled oats
- 1/4 cup chia seeds
- 1/2 cup coconut milk
- 1/4 cup shredded coconut
- 1/4 teaspoon vanilla extract
- Pinch of cinnamon

Instructions:

- In a bowl, combine oats, chia seeds, coconut milk, coconut flakes, and vanilla extract.
- Stir until well combined.
- Let sit for 5-10 minutes, or until thickened.

- Top with cinnamon.

Nutritional Information:

- Calories: approximately 250
- Protein: 5 grams
- Carbohydrates: 35 grams
- Fat: 15 grams

Storage and Reheating:

- Keep leftovers in the fridge for up to three days in an airtight container.
- Reheat until well warmed, either in the stovetop or microwave.

Spinach and Avocado Oatmeal

Yield: 1 serving **Prep Time:** 5 minutes **Cook Time:** 5 minutes

Ingredients:

- 1/4 cup rolled oats
- 1/2 cup spinach
- 1/4 avocado, mashed
- 1/4 cup almond milk
- 1/4 teaspoon lemon juice
- Pinch of salt

Instructions:

- Almond milk and oats should be combined in a small pot. Heat to a simmer on a medium setting.
- Cook for 3-5 minutes, stirring occasionally, until oats are softened.
- Stir in spinach, avocado, lemon juice, and salt.
- Serve immediately.

Nutritional Information:

- Calories: approximately 200
- Protein: 10 grams
- Carbohydrates: 30 grams
- Fat: 10 grams

Storage and Reheating:

- Remaining food can be kept in the fridge for up to three days if it is sealed tightly.
- Warm it again on the stovetop or in the microwave until it's well heated.

Pumpkin Spice Oatmeal

Yield: 1 serving **Prep Time:** 5 minutes **Cook Time:** 5 minutes

Ingredients:

- 1/4 cup rolled oats
- 1/2 cup pumpkin puree
- 1/4 cup almond milk
- 1/4 teaspoon pumpkin pie spice
- Pinch of cinnamon

Instructions:

- Almond milk and oats should be combined in a small pot. Heat to a simmer on a medium setting.
- Cook, stirring periodically, until oats are softened, 3 to 5 minutes.
- Add cinnamon, pumpkin pie spice, and pureed pumpkin.
- Serve immediately.

Nutritional Information:

- Calories: approximately 250
- Protein: 5 grams
- Carbohydrates: 40 grams
- Fat: 10 grams

Storage and Reheating:

- Keep leftovers in the fridge for up to three days in an airtight container.
- Reheat until well warmed, either in the stovetop or microwave.

Tropical Fruit Oatmeal

Yield: 1 serving **Prep Time:** 5 minutes **Cook Time:** 5 minutes

Ingredients:

- 1/4 cup rolled oats
- 1/2 cup tropical fruit mix (mango, pineapple, papaya)
- 1/4 cup coconut milk
- 1 tablespoon honey
- Pinch of cinnamon

Instructions:

- Almond milk and oats should be combined in a small pot. Heat to a simmer on a medium setting.
- Cook for 3-5 minutes, stirring occasionally, until oats are softened.
- Stir in tropical fruit mix, honey, and cinnamon.
- Serve immediately.

Nutritional Information:

- Calories: approximately 250
- Protein: 5 grams
- Carbohydrates: 40 grams
- Fat: 10 grams

Storage and Reheating:

- Keep leftovers in the fridge for up to three days in an airtight container.
- Reheat until well warmed, either in the stovetop or microwave.

<u>Egg Dishes</u>

Scrambled Eggs with Spinach and Tomatoes

Yield: 2 servings Prep Time: 10 minutes Cook Time: 5 minutes

Ingredients:

- 4 large eggs
- 1/2 cup spinach, chopped
- 1/2 cup diced tomatoes
- 1/4 cup chopped scallions
- 1 tablespoon olive oil
- Salt and pepper to taste

Instructions:

- In a medium-size pan, heat the olive oil.
- Cook the spinach and tomatoes until softened.
- In a separate dish, whisk together the eggs.
- Pour the eggs into the skillet and scramble until fully done.
- Add the scallions and season with salt and pepper.
- Serve immediately.

Nutritional Information (per serving):

- Calories: 200-250
- Protein: 15-20g
- Fat: 15-20g
- Carbohydrates: 5-10g

Storage and Reheating:

- Leftovers can be stored in an airtight container in the refrigerator for up to three days.
- Reheating: Reheat gently in a pan or microwave oven.

Avocado Toast with a Poached Egg

Yield: 1 serving Prep Time: 10 minutes Cook Time: 5 minutes

Ingredients:

- 1 slice whole-grain bread
- 1/2 avocado, mashed
- 1 poached egg
- Salt and pepper to taste

Instructions:

- Toast the bread.
- Spread mashed avocado on the toast.

- Top with a poached egg.
- Season with salt and pepper

Nutritional Information (per serving):

- Calories: 300-350
- Fat: 20-25g
- Protein: 15-20g
- Carbohydrates: 20-25g

Storage and Reheating:

- Storage: Store leftover toast in an airtight container in the refrigerator for up to 3 days.
- Reheating: Reheat the toast in a toaster or oven.

Omelet with Vegetables and Herbs

Yield: 1 serving **Prep Time:** 15 minutes **Cook Time:** 5 minutes

Ingredients:

- 2 large eggs
- 1 tablespoon chopped herbs (e.g., parsley, basil)
- 1/2 cup mixed vegetables (e.g., spinach, bell peppers, mushrooms)
- Salt and pepper to taste

Instructions:

- Whisk eggs in a bowl.
- In a pan set over medium heat, sauté veggies.
- Scramble the eggs in the skillet until they are well cooked.
- Season with salt and pepper after adding the herbs.
- Fold the omelet in half.

Nutritional Information (per serving):

- Calories: 200-250
- Fat: 15-20g
- Protein: 15-20g
- Carbohydrates: 5-10g

Storage and Reheating:

- Storage: Refrigerate leftover omelets in an airtight container for up to three days.
- Reheating: Reheat gently in a pan or microwave oven.

Hard-Boiled Eggs with Alkaline-Forming Salad

Yield: 1 serving **Prep Time:** 10 minutes **Cook Time:** 10 minutes

Ingredients:

- 2 large eggs
- 1 cup mixed greens (e.g., spinach, arugula, romaine lettuce)
- 1/2 cup diced cucumbers
- 1/4 cup chopped tomatoes
- 1 tablespoon olive oil
- 1 tablespoon lemon juice
- Salt and pepper to taste

Instructions:

- Hard-boil the eggs.
- In a bowl, combine greens, cucumbers, and tomatoes.
- Add olive oil, lemon juice, salt, and pepper. Toss to coat.
- Peel and chop the hard-boiled eggs.
- Add the chopped eggs to the salad and toss to combine.

Nutritional Information (per serving):

- Calories: 250-300
- Protein: 15-20g
- Fat: 15-20g
- Carbohydrates: 10-15g

Storage and Reheating:

- Refrigerate leftover salad in an airtight container for up to three days.
- Reheating: Reheat the salad gently in a pan or microwave oven.

Chia Seed Pudding with Egg Whites

Yield: 1 serving **Prep Time:** 5 minutes **Cook Time:** None

Ingredients:

- 1/4 cup chia seeds
- 1/2 cup unsweetened almond milk
- 2 egg whites
- 1 tablespoon maple syrup
- 1/4 teaspoon vanilla extract
- Fruit and nuts, for topping

Instructions:

- In a bowl, whisk together chia seeds, almond milk, egg whites, maple syrup, and vanilla extract.
- Cover and refrigerate for at least 30 minutes, or overnight, until the chia seeds have thickened.
- Top with your favorite fruits and nuts.

Nutritional Information (per serving):

- Calories: 200-250
- Protein: 15-20g
- Fat: 10-15g
- Carbohydrates: 20-25g

Storage and Reheating:

- Storage: Refrigerate leftover pudding in an airtight container for up to three days.
- Reheating: If desired, reheat gently in the microwave oven.

Other Options

Quinoa Porridge with Berries and Nuts

Yield: 2 servings **Prep Time:** 10 minutes **Cook Time:** 15 minutes

Ingredients:

- 1/2 cup quinoa, rinsed
- 2 cups water
- 1/4 cup almond milk
- 1/4 cup mixed berries (blueberries, raspberries, strawberries)
- 1/4 cup chopped nuts (almonds, walnuts, pecans)
- Maple syrup (to taste)
- Cinnamon (to taste)

Instructions:

- In a small saucepan, combine quinoa and water. Bring to a boil, then decrease the heat and simmer for 15 minutes, or until the quinoa is cooked.

- Stir in almond milk, berries, nuts, maple syrup, and cinnamon.

- Serve warm and enjoy.

- Calories: 300-350
- Protein: 10-12g
- Carbohydrates: 45-50g
- Fat: 10-12g

Storage and Reheating:

 Store leftovers in an airtight container in the refrigerator for up to 3 days. Reheat in a microwave or saucepan.

Buckwheat Pancakes with Fruit

Yield: 8 pancakes **Prep Time:** 15 minutes **Cook Time:** 20 minutes

Ingredients:

- 1 cup buckwheat flour
- 1/4 cup almond flour
- 2 tablespoons maple syrup
- 1/4 teaspoon baking powder
- 1/4 teaspoon baking soda
- 1/4 teaspoon salt
- 1 cup almond milk
- 1 egg
- 1 tablespoon lemon juice
- 1 tablespoon coconut oil, melted
- Mixed berries (for topping)
- Maple syrup (for topping)

Instructions:

- In a large bowl, whisk together buckwheat flour, almond flour, maple syrup, baking powder, baking soda, and salt.

- In a separate bowl, whisk together almond milk, egg, lemon juice, and melted coconut oil.

- Combine the wet and dry ingredients and whisk until just blended.

- Cook pancakes in a nonstick skillet over medium heat until browned on both sides.

- Serve with mixed berries and maple syrup.

Nutritional Information (per pancake):

- Calories: 150-170

- Protein: 3-4g

- Carbohydrates: 20-25g

- Fat: 5-7g

Leftover pancakes can be stored in an airtight jar in the refrigerator for up to three days. Reheat in a toaster oven or pan.

Hemp Seed Pudding with Coconut Milk

Yield: 2 servings **Prep Time:** 5 minutes **Cook Time:** None

Ingredients:

- 1/4 cup hemp seeds

- 1 cup coconut milk

- 1/4 teaspoon vanilla extract

- 1 tablespoon maple syrup

- 1/4 cup berries (optional)

- Instructions:

- In a small bowl, combine hemp seeds, coconut milk, vanilla extract, and maple syrup.

- Stir well until combined.

- Refrigerate for at least 2 hours, or overnight, to allow the hemp seeds to soften.

- Serve with berries, if desired.

- Calories: 200-220
- Protein: 10-12g
- Carbohydrates: 15-18g
- Fat: 15-18g

Storage and Reheating:

Store leftover pudding in an airtight container in the refrigerator for up to 3 days. Reheat in a microwave or stir into a smoothie.

Alkaline-Forming Granola with Yogurt

Yield: 4 servings **Prep Time:** 20 minutes **Cook Time:** 20 minutes

Ingredients:

- 1 cup rolled oats
- 1/4 cup almond flour
- 1/4 cup chia seeds
- 1/4 cup maple syrup
- 1/4 cup coconut oil, melted
- 1/4 teaspoon cinnamon
- 1/4 teaspoon vanilla extract
- 1/4 cup chopped nuts (almonds, walnuts, pecans)
- 1/2 cup Greek yogurt
- Mixed berries (for topping)

Instructions:

- Preheat oven to 350°F (175°C).
- In a large bowl, combine oats, almond flour, chia seeds, maple syrup, coconut oil, cinnamon, and vanilla extract.
- Mix until well combined.
- Spread the mixture in a baking sheet and bake for 15-20 minutes, or until golden brown.

- Let cool completely, then stir in chopped nuts.

- Serve with Greek yogurt and mixed berries.

Nutritional Information (per serving):

- Calories: 250-270
- Protein: 7-9g

- Carbohydrates: 30-35g
- Fat: 12-14g

Storage and Reheating:

Store leftover granola in an airtight container in the refrigerator for up to 1 week. Reheat in a microwave or toaster oven.

Avocado Toast with Lemon and Herbs

Yield: 2 servings **Prep Time:** 5 minutes **Cook Time:** None

Ingredients:

- 2 slices whole-grain bread
- 1 avocado, mashed
- 1 tablespoon lemon juice

- 1 tablespoon chopped fresh herbs (parsley, dill, cilantro)
- Salt and pepper to taste

Instructions:

- Toast bread slices to your preferred crispiness.
- Spread mashed avocado on top of each slice of toast.
- Drizzle with lemon juice and sprinkle with chopped herbs.
- Season with salt and pepper to taste.

Nutritional Information (per serving):

- Calories: 200-220
- Protein: 3-4g

- Carbohydrates: 25-30g
- Fat: 12-14g

Storage and Reheating: Best enjoyed immediately.

Salads

Kale and Quinoa Salad

Yield: 4 servings **Prep Time:** 30 minutes **Cook Time:** 15 minutes

Ingredients:

- 1 cup cooked quinoa
- 2 cups chopped kale
- 1 cup chopped red onion
- 1/2 cup chopped red bell pepper
- 1/4 cup chopped fresh parsley
- 1/4 cup chopped fresh dill
- 1/4 cup olive oil
- 3 tablespoons lemon juice
- 1 tablespoon maple syrup
- Salt and pepper to taste

Instructions:

- In a large bowl, combine the quinoa, kale, red onion, red bell pepper, parsley, and dill.
- In a small mixing bowl, combine the olive oil, lemon juice, maple syrup, salt, and pepper.
- Toss the salad with the dressing until well coated.
- Serve immediately or refrigerate for later.

Nutritional Information (per serving):

- Calories: 250
- Protein: 7g
- Fat: 15g
- Carbohydrates: 25g

Storage and Reheating:

- Refrigerate leftovers in an airtight jar for up to three days.
- Reheat gently in a pan or microwave.

Avocado and Spinach Salad

Yield: 4 servings **Prep Time:** 20 minutes **Cook Time:** None

Ingredients:

- 2 cups fresh spinach
- 1 avocado, diced
- 1/2 cup chopped red onion
- 1/4 cup chopped red bell pepper
- 1/4 cup crumbled feta cheese
- 1/4 cup olive oil
- 2 tablespoons lemon juice
- Salt and pepper to taste

Instructions:

- In a large mixing bowl, add spinach, avocado, red onion, red bell pepper, and feta cheese.
- In a small mixing bowl, combine the olive oil, lemon juice, salt, and pepper.
- Toss the salad with the dressing until coated.
- Serve immediately.

Nutritional Information (per serving):

- Calories: 200
- Protein: 5g
- Fat: 15g
- Carbohydrates: 10g

Storage and Reheating:

- Refrigerate leftovers in an airtight container for up to one day.
- Do not reheat.

Roasted Vegetable Salad

Yield: 4 servings **Prep Time:** 20 minutes **Cook Time:** 30-40 minutes

Ingredients:

- 1 large, sweet potato, diced
- 1 large zucchini, diced
- 1 large yellow squash, diced
- 1 red onion, cut into wedges
- 1/4 cup olive oil
- 2 tablespoons balsamic vinegar
- 1 teaspoon dried oregano
- 1/2 teaspoon salt
- 1/4 teaspoon black pepper

Instructions:

- Preheat oven to 400°F (200°C).
- In a large mixing bowl, add sweet potato, zucchini, yellow squash, red onion, olive oil, balsamic vinegar, oregano, salt, and pepper. Toss to coat.
- Spread the veggies out in a single layer on a baking sheet.

- Roast for 30 to 40 minutes, or until soft and gently browned.
- Allow to cool somewhat before adding to a salad.

Nutritional Information (per serving):

- Calories: 250
- Protein: 3g
- Fat: 15g
- Carbohydrates: 30g

Storage and Reheating:

- Keep leftovers in an airtight jar in the refrigerator for up to three days.
- Reheat gently in a pan or microwave.

Lentil and Cucumber Salad

Yield: 4 servings **Prep Time:** 20 minutes **Cook Time:** 20-25 minutes

Ingredients:

- 1 cup dried lentils
- 2 cups chopped cucumber
- 1/2 cup chopped red onion
- 1/4 cup chopped fresh mint
- 1/4 cup olive oil
- 2 tablespoons lemon juice
- 1 garlic clove, minced
- Salt and pepper to taste

Instructions:

- Cook the lentils according to package directions.
- In a large mixing dish, add cooked lentils, cucumber, red onion, and mint.
- In a small bowl, combine the olive oil, lemon juice, garlic, salt, and pepper.
- Toss the salad with the dressing until well coated.
- Serve immediately or refrigerate for later.

Nutritional Information (per serving):

Calories: 200

Protein: 10g

Fat: 10g

Carbohydrates: 25g

Storage and Reheating:

- Refrigerate leftovers in an airtight jar for up to three days.
- Reheat gently in a pan or microwave.

Beetroot and Goat Cheese Salad

Yield: 4 servings **Prep Time:** 20 minutes **Cook Time:** 0 minutes

Ingredients:

- 1 cup cooked beets, diced
- 1 cup chopped spinach
- 1/2 cup crumbled goat cheese
- 1/4 cup chopped walnuts
- 1/4 cup olive oil
- 2 tablespoons balsamic vinegar
- 1 garlic clove, minced
- Salt and pepper to taste

Instructions:

- In a large bowl, combine the beets, spinach, goat cheese, and walnuts.
- In a small bowl, combine olive oil, balsamic vinegar, garlic, salt, and pepper.
- Toss the salad with the dressing until well coated.
- Serve immediately.

Nutritional Information (per serving):

- Calories: 250
- Protein: 10g
- Fat: 15g
- Carbohydrates: 15g

Storage and Reheating:

- Refrigerate leftovers in an airtight jar for up to two days.
- Do not reheat.

Bowls recipes

Buddha Bowl

Yield: 2 servings **Prep Time:** 15 minutes **Cook Time:** 10 minutes

Ingredients:

- 1 cup cooked quinoa or brown rice
- One cup of roasted veggies, such as sweet potatoes, carrots, and broccoli
- 1/2 cup cooked protein (e.g., tofu, chickpeas, grilled chicken)
- 1/4 cup chopped nuts or seeds (e.g., almonds, sunflower seeds)
- 1/4 cup fresh herbs (e.g., cilantro, parsley)
- 1/4 cup dressing (e.g., lemon-tahini dressing)

Instructions:

- Combine cooked quinoa or brown rice, roasted vegetables, protein, nuts or seeds, and herbs in a bowl.
- Drizzle with dressing and toss to coat.

Nutritional Information:

- Calories: Approximately 500-600 per serving
- Protein: 20-25 grams per serving
- Carbohydrates: 50-60 grams per serving
- Fat: 20-25 grams per serving

Storage and Reheating:

- Remaining food can be kept in the refrigerator for up to three days if it is sealed tightly.
- Reheat in the oven or microwave until well warm.

Power Bowl

Yield: 2 servings Prep Time: 15 minutes Cook Time: 10 minutes

Ingredients:

- 1 cup cooked quinoa or brown rice
- 1 cup roasted vegetables (e.g., Brussels sprouts, sweet potatoes, red peppers)
- 1/2 cup cooked protein (e.g., salmon, lentils, chickpeas)
- 1/4 cup chopped nuts or seeds (e.g., walnuts, pumpkin seeds)
- 1/4 cup fresh herbs (e.g., basil, mint)
- 1/4 cup dressing (e.g., avocado-lime dressing)

Instructions:

- Combine cooked quinoa or brown rice, roasted vegetables, protein, nuts or seeds, and herbs in a bowl.
- Drizzle with dressing and toss to coat.

Nutritional Information:

- Calories: Approximately 500-600 per serving
- Protein: 20-25 grams per serving
- Carbohydrates: 50-60 grams per serving
- Fat: 20-25 grams per serving

Storage and Reheating:

- Keep leftovers in the fridge for up to three days in an airtight container.
- Use a microwave or oven to reheat until well hot.

Grain Bowl

Yield: 2 servings **Prep Time:** 15 minutes **Cook Time:** 10 minutes

Ingredients:

- 1 cup cooked grain of your choice (e.g., quinoa, brown rice, farro)
- 1 cup roasted vegetables (e.g., asparagus, zucchini, bell peppers)
- 1/2 cup cooked protein (e.g., tofu, tempeh, grilled chicken)
- 1/4 cup chopped nuts or seeds (e.g., almonds, sunflower seeds)
- 1/4 cup fresh herbs (e.g., cilantro, parsley)
- 1/4 cup dressing (e.g., tahini-ginger dressing)

Instructions:

- Combine cooked grain, roasted vegetables, protein, nuts or seeds, and herbs in a bowl.
- Drizzle with dressing and toss to coat.

Nutritional Information:

- Calories: Approximately 500-600 per serving
- Protein: 20-25 grams per serving
- Carbohydrates: 50-60 grams per serving
- Fat: 20-25 grams per serving

Storage and Reheating:

- Keep leftovers in the fridge for up to three days in an airtight container.
- Use a microwave or oven to reheat until well hot.

Salad Bowl

Yield: 2 servings **Prep Time:** 15 minutes **Cook Time:** N/A

Ingredients:

- 1 cup mixed greens
- 1/2 cup chopped vegetables (e.g., cucumber, tomato, bell pepper)
- 1/4 cup cooked protein (e.g., grilled chicken, tofu, chickpeas)
- 1/4 cup chopped nuts or seeds (e.g., walnuts, pumpkin seeds)
- 1/4 cup dressing (e.g., lemon-dill dressing)

Instructions:

- Combine mixed greens, vegetables, protein, nuts or seeds in a bowl.
- Drizzle with dressing and toss to coat.

Nutritional Information:

- Calories: Approximately 300-400 per serving
- Protein: 15-20 grams per serving
- Carbohydrates: 30-40 grams per serving
- Fat: 15-20 grams per serving

Storage and Reheating:

- Keep leftovers in the fridge for up to three days in an airtight container.
- Use a microwave or oven to reheat until well hot.

Smoothie Bowl

Yield: 1 serving **Prep Time:** 5 minutes **Cook Time:** N/A

Ingredients:

- 1 cup frozen fruit (e.g., berries, mango, banana)
- 1/2 cup plant-based milk (e.g., almond milk, coconut milk)
- 1 tablespoon chia seeds or hemp seeds
- 1 tablespoon protein powder (optional)
- Toppings: fresh fruit, nuts, seeds, granola, honey

Instructions:

- Blend frozen fruit, plant-based milk, chia seeds, and protein powder until smooth.
- Pour into a bowl and top with desired toppings.

Nutritional Information:

- Calories: Approximately 300-400 per serving
- Protein: 15-20 grams per serving
- Carbohydrates: 40-50 grams per serving
- Fat: 10-15 grams per serving

Storage and Reheating:

- Smoothie bowls are best consumed fresh. If storing leftovers, cover tightly and refrigerate for up to 1 day.
- Reheat in a microwave or blend with additional liquid if desired.

Spinach and Feta Wrap

Yield: 2 servings **Prep Time:** 15 minutes **Cook Time:** 5 minutes

Ingredients:

- 2 large whole-wheat tortillas
- 1 cup cooked spinach
- 1/2 cup crumbled feta cheese
- 1/4 cup diced red onion
- 1/4 cup diced cucumber
- 2 tablespoons balsamic vinegar
- 1 tablespoon olive oil

Instructions:

- In a bowl, combine the spinach, feta cheese, red onion, and cucumber.
- Drizzle with balsamic vinegar and olive oil and toss to coat.
- Place the spinach mixture on one side of a tortilla.
- Tightly roll up the tortilla by folding its edges over the contents.
- Continue with the other tortilla.
- You can either serve it right away or keep it in the fridge for up to two days.

Nutritional Information (per serving):

- Calories: 250
- Protein: 15g
- Fat: 12g
- Carbohydrates: 25g

Storage and Reheating:

- Remaining food can be kept in the fridge for up to two days.
- Reheat the wrap by covering it with foil and heating it for ten to fifteen minutes at 350°F (175°C) in a preheated oven.

Hummus and Veggie Wrap

Yield: 2 servings **Prep Time:** 15 minutes **Cook Time:** 0 minutes

Ingredients:

- 2 large whole-wheat tortillas
- 1/2 cup hummus
- 1/4 cup diced red onion
- 1/4 cup diced cucumber
- 1/4 cup diced bell pepper
- 1/4 cup diced tomato
- 1 tablespoon lemon juice

Instructions:

- Spread hummus on one side of a tortilla.
- Top with red onion, cucumber, bell pepper, and tomato.
- Drizzle with lemon juice.
- Roll up tightly.
- Repeat with the second tortilla.
- You can either serve it right away or keep it in the fridge for up to two days.

- Calories: 200
- Protein: 10g
- Fat: 10g
- Carbohydrates: 25g

Storage and Reheating:

- Store leftovers in the refrigerator for up to 2 days.
- To reheat, wrap the wrap in foil and warm in a preheated oven at 350°F (175°C) for 10-15 minutes.

Avocado and Tomato Wrap

Yield: 2 servings **Prep Time:** 10 minutes **Cook Time:** 0 minutes

Ingredients:

- 2 large whole-wheat tortillas
- 1/2 avocado, mashed
- 1/4 cup diced tomato
- 1/4 cup diced red onion
- 1 tablespoon lemon juice
- 1 teaspoon cumin

Instructions:

- Spread mashed avocado on one side of a tortilla.
- Top with tomato and red onion.
- Pour some lemon juice over it and then add some cumin.
- Roll up tightly.
- Repeat with the second tortilla.
- You can either serve it right away or keep it in the fridge for up to two days.

Nutritional Information (per serving):

- Calories: 250
- Protein: 5g
- Fat: 15g
- Carbohydrates: 25g

Storage and Reheating:

- Remaining food can be kept in the fridge for up to two days.

- Reheat the wrap by covering it with foil and heating it for ten to fifteen minutes at 350°F (175°C) in a preheated oven.

Lentil and Quinoa Wrap

Yield: 2 servings Prep Time: 20 minutes Cook Time: 20 minutes

Ingredients:

- 2 large whole-wheat tortillas
- 1 cup cooked lentils
- 1/2 cup cooked quinoa
- 1/4 cup diced red onion
- 1/4 cup diced bell pepper
- 1/4 cup diced cucumber
- 1 tablespoon olive oil
- 1 teaspoon cumin

Instructions:

- In a bowl, combine the lentils, quinoa, red onion, bell pepper, and cucumber.
- Coat in olive oil and season with cumin.
- Spoon mixture onto one tortilla's side.
- Tightly roll.
- After that, repeat with the second tortilla.
- Serve right away or keep chilled for up to two days.

Nutritional Information (per serving):

- Calories: 300
- Protein: 20g
- Fat: 10g
- Carbohydrates: 35g

Storage and Reheating:

- Remaining food can be kept in the fridge for up to two days.
- Reheat the wrap by covering it with foil and heating it for ten to fifteen minutes at 350°F (175°C) in a preheated oven.

Grilled Vegetable Wrap

Yield: 2 servings Prep Time: 15 minutes Cook Time: 15 minutes

Ingredients:

- 2 large whole-wheat tortillas
- 1 red bell pepper, sliced
- 1 yellow bell pepper, sliced
- 1 zucchini, sliced
- 1 squash, sliced
- 1 tablespoon olive oil
- 1/4 cup hummus
- 1/4 cup diced cucumber

Instructions:

- Preheat grill to medium-high heat.
- Brush the vegetables with olive oil and grill for 5-7 minutes per side, or until tender.
- Spread hummus on one side of a tortilla.
- Top with grilled vegetables and cucumber.
- Roll up tightly.
- Repeat with the second tortilla.
- You can either serve it right away or keep it in the fridge for up to two days.

Nutritional Information (per serving):

- Calories: 250
- Protein: 10g
- Fat: 15g
- Carbohydrates: 25g

Storage and Reheating:

- Remaining food can be kept in the fridge for up to two days.
- Reheat the wrap by covering it with foil and heating it for ten to fifteen minutes at 350°F (175°C) in a preheated oven.

Soups

Lentil Soup

Yield: 4 servings Prep Time: 15 minutes Cook Time: 30 minutes

Ingredients:

- 1 cup dried brown lentils
- 1 onion, chopped
- 2 carrots, chopped
- 2 celery stalks, chopped
- 4 cloves garlic, minced
- 1 teaspoon dried thyme
- 1 teaspoon dried rosemary
- 1/2 teaspoon red pepper flakes
- 4 cups vegetable broth
- 1 can (15 ounces) diced tomatoes
- Salt and pepper to taste

Instructions:

- Rinse the lentils and set aside.
- Add the onion, carrots, celery, and garlic to a large saucepan and sauté until softened.
- Add the lentils, thyme, rosemary, red pepper flakes, vegetable broth, and diced tomatoes to the pot.

- Bring to a boil, then decrease the heat and simmer for 30 minutes, or until the lentils are cooked.
- Season with salt and pepper to taste.

Nutritional Information (per serving):

- Calories: 250
- Protein: 15g
- Fat: 5g
- Carbohydrates: 35g

Storage and Reheating:

- Keep leftovers in the fridge for up to three days in an airtight container.
- Warm up slowly in the microwave or on the stovetop.

Vegetable Soup

Yield: 6 servings **Prep Time:** 20 minutes **Cook Time:** 30 minutes

Ingredients:

- 1 tablespoon olive oil
- 1 onion, chopped
- 2 carrots, chopped
- 2 celery stalks, chopped
- 4 cloves garlic, minced
- 1 potato, cubed
- 1 can (15 ounces) chickpeas
- 1 can (15 ounces) diced tomatoes
- 4 cups vegetable broth
- 1 bay leaf
- Salt and pepper to taste

Instructions:

- In a big saucepan set over medium heat, warm the olive oil.
- When they start to soften, add the onion, carrots, celery, and garlic.
- Incorporate the bay leaf, potatoes, chickpeas, tomatoes, and vegetable broth.
- Once the veggies are soft, bring to a boil, lower the heat, and simmer for 30 minutes.
- After removing the bay leaf, add salt and pepper to taste.

Nutritional Information (per serving):

- Calories: 200
- Protein: 10g
- Fat: 5g
- Carbohydrates: 30g

Storage and Reheating:

- Keep leftovers in the fridge for up to three days in an airtight container.
- Reheat gently on the stovetop or in the microwave.

Tomato Soup

Yield: 4 servings **Prep Time:** 15 minutes **Cook Time:** 25 minutes

Ingredients:

- 2 tablespoons olive oil
- 1 onion, chopped
- 2 cloves garlic, minced
- 1 can (28 ounces) diced tomatoes
- 4 cups vegetable broth
- 1 bay leaf
- 1/2 teaspoon dried oregano
- 1/4 teaspoon red pepper flakes
- Salt and pepper to taste

Instructions:

- In a big saucepan set over medium heat, warm the olive oil.
- Add the garlic and onion and sauté until tender.
- Incorporate the chopped tomatoes, veggie stock, bay leaf, oregano, and red chili powder.
- Bring to a boil, then reduce heat and simmer for 25 minutes, or until the flavors have blended.
- Remove the bay leaf and puree the soup using a blender or immersion blender.
- Season with salt and pepper to taste.

Nutritional Information (per serving):

- Calories: 150
- Protein: 5g
- Fat: 3g
- Carbohydrates: 25g

Storage and Reheating:

- Refrigerate leftovers in an airtight jar for up to three days.
- Reheat gently on the stovetop or in the microwave.

Broccoli Cheddar Soup

Yield: 4 servings **Prep Time:** 15 minutes **Cook Time:** 30 minutes

Ingredients:

- 1 tablespoon butter
- 1 onion, chopped
- 2 cloves garlic, minced
- 1 head of broccoli, chopped
- 4 cups vegetable broth
-
- 1/2 cup all-purpose flour
- 1 cup milk
- 1 cup shredded cheddar cheese
- Salt and pepper to taste

Instructions:

- In a large saucepan over medium heat, melt the butter.
- Cook the garlic and onion until they become tender.
- Bring the vegetable broth and broccoli to a boil after adding them.

- Simmer the broccoli over low heat until it becomes soft.
- Mix the flour and milk together in another basin until they are well combined.
- Stir the flour mixture into the soup gradually until it thickens.
- Add the shredded cheddar cheese and stir until it melts.
- Season with salt and pepper to taste.

Nutritional Information (per serving):

- Calories: 250
- Protein: 10g
- Fat: 15g
- Carbohydrates: 20g

Storage and Reheating:

- Refrigerate leftovers in an airtight jar for up to three days.
- Reheat gently on the stovetop or in the microwave.

Coconut Curry Soup

Yield: 4 servings **Prep Time:** 15 minutes **Cook Time:** 30 minutes

Ingredients:

- 1 tablespoon coconut oil
- 1 onion, chopped
- 2 cloves garlic, minced
- 1 can (15 ounces) chickpeas
- 1 can (15 ounces) diced tomatoes
- 1 can (14.5 ounces) coconut milk
- 1 tablespoon curry powder
- 1 teaspoon ground cumin
- 1/2 teaspoon red pepper flakes
- Salt and pepper to taste

Instructions:

- In a large saucepan, warm the coconut oil over medium heat.
- Add the onion and garlic and cook until softened.
- Add the chickpeas, diced tomatoes, coconut milk, curry powder, cumin, and red pepper flakes.
- Bring to a boil, then reduce heat and simmer for 30 minutes, or until the flavors have blended.
- Season with salt and pepper to taste.

Nutritional Information (per serving):

Calories: 250

Protein: 15g

Fat: 10g

Carbohydrates: 25g

Storage and Reheating:

- Refrigerate leftovers in an airtight jar for up to three days.
- Reheat gently on the stovetop or in the microwave

Vegetable-Based

Roasted Vegetable Medley with Quinoa

Yield: 4 servings **Prep Time:** 20 minutes **Cook Time:** 30-35 minutes

Ingredients:

- 1 cup quinoa, cooked
- 1 large, sweet potato, cubed
- 1 red onion, quartered
- 1 red bell pepper, cut into strips
- 1 zucchini, diced
- 1 cup Brussels sprouts, halved
- 2 tablespoons olive oil
- 1 teaspoon dried oregano
- 1/2 teaspoon salt
- 1/4 teaspoon black pepper

Instructions:

- Preheat oven to 400°F (200°C).
- In a large bowl, combine sweet potato, red onion, bell pepper, zucchini, Brussels sprouts, olive oil, oregano, salt, and pepper. Toss to coat.
- Spread the vegetable mixture on a baking sheet lined with parchment paper.
- Roast for 30-35 minutes, or until vegetables are tender and slightly browned.
- Serve the roasted vegetables over cooked quinoa

Nutritional Information (per serving):

- Calories: 300-350
- Protein: 10-12 grams
- Carbohydrates: 35-40 grams
- Fat: 15-18 grams

Leftovers may be refrigerated in an airtight container for up to three days and reheated in the microwave or oven.

Spinach and Feta Salad with Lemon Vinaigrette

Yield: 4 servings **Prep Time:** 15 minutes

Ingredients:

- 1 bunch fresh spinach
- 1 cup crumbled feta cheese
- 1/2 cup cherry tomatoes, halved
- 1/4 cup red onion, thinly sliced
- 1/4 cup cucumber, diced

For the vinaigrette:

- 1/4 cup olive oil
- 1/4 cup lemon juice
- 1 tablespoon honey
- 1/2 teaspoon Dijon mustard
- Salt and pepper to taste

Instructions:

- In a large bowl, combine spinach, feta cheese, cherry tomatoes, red onion, and cucumber.
- In a small bowl, whisk together olive oil, lemon juice, honey, Dijon mustard, salt, and pepper to make the vinaigrette.
- Toss the salad with the vinaigrette until well coated.

Nutritional Information (per serving):

- Calories: 200-220
- Protein: 10-12 grams
- Carbohydrates: 15-18 grams
- Fat: 15-18 grams

Storage: Store leftovers in an airtight container in the refrigerator for up to 2 days.

Grilled Zucchini and Squash with Avocado Pesto

Yield: 4 servings **Prep Time:** 15 minutes **Cook Time:** 15-20 minutes

Ingredients:

- 2 zucchinis, sliced lengthwise
- 2 squashes, sliced lengthwise
- 1/4 cup olive oil
- 1/4 cup lemon juice
- Salt and pepper to taste

For the pesto:

- 1 cup fresh basil leaves
- 1/2 cup pine nuts
- 1/4 cup grated Parmesan cheese
- 1/4 cup olive oil
- 1 clove garlic, minced
- Salt and pepper to taste

Instructions:

- Preheat grill to medium-high heat.
- In a small mixing dish, combine olive oil, lemon juice, salt, and pepper. Brush the zucchini and squash slices with the mixture.
- Grill the zucchini and squash for 15-20 minutes, or until tender and slightly charred.
- While the zucchini and squash are grilling, prepare the pesto by combining basil, pine nuts, Parmesan cheese, olive oil, garlic, salt, and pepper in a food processor. Pulse until smooth.
- Serve the grilled zucchini and squash with the avocado pesto.

Nutritional Information (per serving):

- Calories: 250-270
- Protein: 4-5 grams
- Carbohydrates: 15-18 grams
- Fat: 20-22 grams

Storage: Store leftovers in an airtight container in the refrigerator for up to 2 days. Reheat on the grill or in the oven.

Cauliflower Steak with Lemon-Herb Sauce

Yield: 4 servings **Prep Time:** 15 minutes **Cook Time:** 20-25 minutes

Ingredients:

- One big head of cauliflower, sliced into steaks
- 1 tablespoon olive oil
- 1/2 teaspoon salt
- 1/4 teaspoon black pepper

For the sauce:

- 1/4 cup lemon juice
- 2 tablespoons olive oil
- 1 clove garlic, minced
- 1 teaspoon dried thyme
- 1/2 teaspoon dried oregano
- Salt and pepper to taste

Instructions:

- Preheat grill to medium-high heat.
- Add salt and pepper to the cauliflower steaks after brushing them with olive oil.
- The cauliflower steaks should be soft and faintly browned after 20 to 25 minutes on the grill.
- While the cauliflower is grilling, prepare the sauce by combining lemon juice, olive oil, garlic, thyme, oregano, salt, and pepper in a small bowl.
- Serve the grilled cauliflower steaks with the lemon-herb sauce.

Nutritional Information (per serving):

- Calories: 150-170
- Protein: 5-7 grams
- Carbohydrates: 15-18 grams
- Fat: 10-12 grams

Storage: Remaining food can be kept in the fridge for up to two days if it is sealed tightly. Warm through in the oven or on the grill.

Walnuts and goat cheese in a roasted beet salad

Yield: 4 servings Prep Time: 15 minutes Cook Time: 30-35 minutes

Ingredients:

- 2 beets, peeled and quartered
- 1 tablespoon olive oil
- 1/2 teaspoon salt
- 1/4 teaspoon black pepper
- 1/2 cup crumbled goat cheese
- 1/4 cup walnuts, toasted
- 1/4 cup mixed greens
- 1/4 cup balsamic vinaigrette

Instructions:

- Preheat oven to 400°F (200°C).
- Mix the beets with salt, pepper, and olive oil.
- After roasting for 30 to 35 minutes, the beets should be soft.
- Slice the beets into wedges after allowing them to cool somewhat.
- In a large bowl, combine the roasted beets, goat cheese, walnuts, mixed greens, and balsamic vinaigrette. Toss to coat.

Green Bean and Potato Casserole

Yield: 4 servings **Prep Time:** 30 minutes **Cook Time:** 30 minutes

Ingredients:

- 1-pound green beans, trimmed
- 2 large potatoes, peeled and cubed
- 1 onion, chopped
- 2 cloves garlic, minced
- 1 cup vegetable broth
- 1/2 cup grated Parmesan cheese
- 1/4 cup breadcrumbs
- 2 tablespoons butter, melted
- Salt and pepper to taste

Instructions:

- Preheat oven to 375°F (190°C).
- In a large saucepan, bring vegetable broth to a boil. Add green beans and potatoes and cook until tender. Drain.
- In a large bowl, combine cooked vegetables, onion, garlic, Parmesan cheese, breadcrumbs, melted butter, salt, and pepper.
- Pour the mixture into a casserole dish that has been oiled, and bake for 30 minutes, or until bubbling and golden brown.

Nutritional Information (per serving):

- Calories: 250
- Protein: 10g
- Fat: 12g
- Carbohydrates: 25g

Storage and Reheating:

- Remaining food can be kept in the refrigerator for up to three days if it is sealed tightly.
- Reheat in a covered dish in the oven at 350°F (175°C) for 20-25 minutes.

Asparagus and Salmon Salad with Lemon-Dill Dressing

Yield: 4 servings **Prep Time:** 20 minutes **Cook Time:** 10-12 minutes

Ingredients:

- 1 pound asparagus, trimmed
- 1 pound salmon fillets
- 1/2 cup lemon juice
- 1/4 cup olive oil
- 2 tablespoons fresh dill, chopped
- Salt and pepper to taste

Instructions:

- Preheat grill or broiler.
- Toss asparagus with olive oil, salt, and pepper. Grill or broil until tender-crisp.
- Season salmon fillets with salt and pepper. Grill or broil until cooked through.
- In a small bowl, whisk together lemon juice, olive oil, and dill.
- Arrange grilled asparagus and salmon on a serving platter.
- Drizzle with lemon-dill dressing.

Nutritional Information (per serving):

- Calories: 400
- Protein: 30g
- Fat: 25g
- Carbohydrates: 10g

Storage and Reheating:

- Keep leftovers in the fridge for up to two days in an airtight container.
- Reheat salmon and asparagus separately on the grill or in the oven.

Stir-Fried Vegetables with Tofu

Yield: 4 servings **Prep Time:** 15 minutes **Cook Time:** 15 minutes

Ingredients:

- 1 pound mixed vegetables (broccoli, carrots, bell peppers, onions)
- 1 block extra-firm tofu, pressed and cubed
- 2 tablespoons soy sauce

- 1 tablespoon rice vinegar
- 1 teaspoon sesame oil
- 1 clove garlic, minced
- Salt and pepper to taste

Instructions:

- Heat a large skillet over medium-high heat. Add a tablespoon of oil.
- Tofu cubes should be added and cooked until browned all over.
- Add chopped vegetables and stir-fry until tender-crisp.
- Stir in soy sauce, rice vinegar, sesame oil, and garlic.
- Season with salt and pepper to taste.

Nutritional Information (per serving):

- Calories: 250
- Protein: 20g
- Fat: 10g
- Carbohydrates: 20g

Storage and Reheating:

- The remaining food can be kept in the fridge for up to three days if it is sealed tightly.
- Reheat in a skillet over medium heat.

Roasted Vegetable Soup with Coconut Milk

Yield: 4 servings **Prep Time:** 20 minutes **Cook Time:** 30 minutes

Ingredients:

- 1 tablespoon olive oil
- 1 onion, chopped
- 2 carrots, chopped
- 2 celery stalks, chopped
- 2 cloves garlic, minced
- 1 butternut squash, peeled and cubed
- 4 cups vegetable broth
- 1 can (14.5 oz) coconut milk
- Salt and pepper to taste

Instructions:

- Preheat oven to 400°F (200°C).
- Mix olive oil, salt, and pepper with butternut squash. Roast until soft.

- In a big saucepan set over medium heat, warm the olive oil. Cook the onion, carrots, and celery until they become tender.
- Add the garlic and heat for a further minute.
- Incorporate the roasted butternut squash, coconut milk, and vegetable broth. Once the veggies are soft, bring to a boil, lower the heat, and simmer for 15 to 20 minutes.
- Puree soup with an immersion blender or in a blender. Season with salt and pepper to taste.

Nutritional Information (per serving):

- Calories: 250
- Protein: 5g
- Fat: 15g
- Carbohydrates: 25g

Storage and Reheating:

- Refrigerate leftovers in an airtight container for up to 3 days.
- Reheat over medium heat, stirring often.

Lentil and Vegetable Curry

Yield: 4 servings **Prep Time:** 30 minutes **Cook Time:** 30 minutes

Ingredients:

- 1 cup dried red lentils
- 1 onion, chopped
- 2 cloves garlic, minced
- 1 teaspoon ground cumin
- 1 teaspoon ground coriander
- 1/2 teaspoon turmeric
- 1 can (14.5 oz) diced tomatoes
- 1 can (15 oz) coconut milk
- 1 cup vegetable broth
- 1 cup mixed vegetables (broccoli, carrots, bell peppers)
- Salt and pepper to taste

Instructions:

- Rinse lentils and set aside.
- In a large saucepan, heat the olive oil over medium heat. Cook the onion and garlic until softened.
- Stir in cumin, coriander, and turmeric. Cook for 1 minute more.

- Add diced tomatoes, coconut milk, vegetable broth, and lentils. Bring to a boil, then decrease the heat and simmer for 20-25 minutes, or until the lentils are cooked.
- Stir in mixed vegetables and cook for 5-7 minutes more, or until vegetables are tender-crisp.
- Season with salt and pepper to taste.

Nutritional Information (per serving):

- Calories: 300
- Protein: 15g
- Fat: 15g
- Carbohydrates: 30g

Storage and Reheating:

- Refrigerate leftovers in an airtight jar for up to three days.
- Reheat on the stovetop over medium heat, stirring occasionally.

Protein-Packed:

Grilled Salmon with Roasted Vegetables

Yield: 4 servings **Prep Time:** 20 minutes **Cook Time:** 15-20 minutes

Ingredients:

- 4 salmon fillets (6 oz each)
- 1 tablespoon olive oil
- 1 teaspoon lemon zest
- 1 tablespoon lemon juice
- 1/2 teaspoon garlic powder
- 1/4 teaspoon salt
- 1/4 teaspoon black pepper
- 1 large, sweet potato, cubed
- 1 red bell pepper, cut into strips
- 1 zucchini, cut into rounds
- 1 tablespoon olive oil
- 1/2 teaspoon dried oregano
- 1/4 teaspoon salt
- 1/4 teaspoon black pepper

Instructions:

- Preheat grill to medium-high heat.
- In a small bowl, combine olive oil, lemon zest, lemon juice, garlic powder, salt, and pepper. Brush salmon fillets with the marinade.

- Toss sweet potato, bell pepper, zucchini, olive oil, oregano, salt, and pepper in a bowl.
- Grill salmon for 15-20 minutes, or until cooked through.
- Grill vegetables for 10-12 minutes, or until tender-crisp.
- Serve salmon with roasted vegetables.

- Calories: 350-400
- Protein: 30-35g
- Carbohydrates: 25-30g
- Fat: 20-25g

Refrigerate leftovers in an airtight jar for up to three days. Reheat in a preheated oven at 350°F (175°C) for 10-15 minutes.

Chicken Breast with Lemon-Herb Marinade and Steamed Broccoli

Yield: 4 servings Prep Time: 20 minutes Cook Time: 20-25 minutes

Ingredients:

- 4 boneless, skinless chicken breasts
- 1/4 cup olive oil
- 1/4 cup lemon juice
- 2 cloves garlic, minced
- 1 teaspoon dried oregano
- 1/2 teaspoon dried thyme
- 1/4 teaspoon salt
- 1/4 teaspoon black pepper
- 1 head broccoli, cut into florets

Instructions:

- In a mixing bowl, add olive oil, lemon juice, garlic, oregano, thyme, salt, and pepper.
- Add chicken breasts to the marinade and let them sit for at least 30 minutes, or up to 4 hours.
- Steam broccoli until tender-crisp.
- Grill or bake chicken breasts until cooked through.
- Serve chicken with steamed broccoli.

Nutritional Information (per serving):

- Calories: 250-300
- Protein: 30-35g
- Carbohydrates: 10-15g
- Fat: 15-20g

Refrigerate leftovers in an airtight jar for up to three days. Reheat in a preheated oven at 350°F (175°C) for 10-15 minutes.

Tofu Scramble with Spinach and Tomatoes

Yield: 4 servings Prep Time: 15 minutes Cook Time: 10-12 minutes

Ingredients:

- 1 block extra-firm tofu, crumbled
- 1 tablespoon olive oil
- 1/2 onion, chopped
- 2 cloves garlic, minced
- 1 cup spinach
- 1 tomato, diced
- 1/4 cup nutritional yeast
- 1 tablespoon tamari
- 1/4 teaspoon salt
- 1/4 teaspoon black pepper

Instructions:

- In a large skillet, heat the olive oil over medium heat.
- Cook the onion and garlic until they are softened.
- Add crumbled tofu and cook for 5-7 minutes, or until heated through.
- Stir in spinach and tomato and cook until spinach wilts.
- Season with nutritional yeast, tamari, salt, and pepper.

Nutritional Information (per serving):

- Calories: 200-250
- Protein: 20-25g
- Carbohydrates: 10-15g
- Fat: 10-15g

Refrigerate leftovers in an airtight jar for up to three days. Reheat in a skillet over medium heat.

Shrimp Scampi with Zucchini Noodles

Yield: 4 servings Prep Time: 15 minutes Cook Time: 15-20 minutes

Ingredients:

- 1-pound large shrimp, peeled and deveined
- 2 cloves garlic, minced
- 1/4 cup white wine
- 1/4 cup lemon juice
- 1/4 cup butter
- 1/4 cup grated Parmesan cheese
- 2 zucchinis, spiralized into noodles

- 1/4 teaspoon red pepper flakes (optional)

Instructions:

- In a large skillet, melt butter over medium-high heat.
- Cook for 30 seconds, or until the garlic is aromatic.
- Add the shrimp and heat for 2-3 minutes per side, or until done.
- Deglaze the skillet with white wine and lemon juice.
- Mix in the Parmesan cheese and red pepper flakes (if using).
- Add zucchini noodles and toss to coat.

Nutritional Information (per serving):

- Calories: 250-300
- Carbohydrates: 10-15g
- Protein: 25-30g
- Fat: 15-20g

Leftovers can be stored in an airtight container in the refrigerator for up to three days. Rewarm in a skillet over medium heat.

Turkey Burgers with Avocado Mayo and Sweet Potato Fries

Yield: 4 servings Prep Time: 20 minutes Cook Time: 20-25 minutes

Ingredients:

- 1 pound ground turkey
- 1/4 teaspoon black pepper
- 1/2 cup breadcrumbs
- 1 large, sweet potato, cut into fries
- 1/4 cup finely chopped onion
- 1/4 cup avocado, mashed
- 1 egg, beaten
- 1 tablespoon lemon juice
- 1 tablespoon Dijon mustard
- 1 clove garlic, minced
- 1/4 teaspoon salt

Instructions:

- Preheat grill or skillet to medium-high heat.
- In a bowl, combine ground turkey, breadcrumbs, onion, egg, Dijon mustard, salt, and pepper. Shape into 4 patties.

- Grill or cook patties for 15-20 minutes, or until cooked through.

- Bake sweet potato fries in a preheated oven at 400°F (200°C) for 20-25 minutes, or until crispy.

- To make avocado mayo, combine avocado, lemon juice, and garlic.

- Serve the turkey burgers with avocado mayo and sweet potato fries.

- Calories: 350-400
- Carbohydrates: 30-35g
- Protein: 30-35g
- Fat: 15-20g

Leftovers can be refrigerated in an airtight container for up to three days. Reheat the mixture in a skillet over medium heat.

Baked Chicken Breast with Roasted Brussels Sprouts

Yield: 4 servings Prep Time: 15 minutes Cook Time: 30-35 minutes

Ingredients:

- 2 boneless, skinless chicken breasts
- 2 tablespoons olive oil
- 1 tablespoon olive oil
- 1/4 teaspoon garlic powder
- Salt and pepper to taste
- 1/4 teaspoon red pepper flakes
- 1 pound Brussels sprouts, trimmed and halved

Instructions:

- Preheat oven to 400°F (200°C).
- Season chicken breasts with salt and pepper.
- Drizzle chicken breasts with olive oil and arrange them on a baking pan.
- Roast for a total of 25 to 30 minutes, or until done.
- Toss Brussels sprouts with olive oil, garlic powder, and red pepper flakes.
- Place Brussels sprouts on a baking sheet and roast for 20-25 minutes, or until tender.
- Serve chicken breasts with roasted Brussels sprouts.

Nutritional Information (per serving):

- Calories: 350-400
- Protein: 40-45 grams
- Carbohydrates: 15-20 grams
- Fat: 15-20 grams

Storage: Keep leftovers in the fridge for up to three days in an airtight container.

Reheating: Reheat leftovers in the oven at 350°F (175°C) until heated through.

Fish Tacos with Avocado Salsa and Lime Crema

Yield: 4 servings **Prep Time:** 30 minutes **Cook Time:** 10-15 minutes

Ingredients:

- 1-pound white fish fillets (e.g., cod, tilapia)
- 1 tablespoon olive oil
- Salt and pepper to taste
- 8 corn tortillas
- 1 avocado, diced
- 1 tomato, diced
- 1/2 red onion, diced
- 1 lime, juiced
- 1/4 cup cilantro, chopped
- 1/4 cup Greek yogurt
- 1 tablespoon lime juice
- 1/4 teaspoon cumin

Instructions:

- Season fish fillets with salt and pepper.
- In a pan set over medium-high heat, warm the olive oil.
- Cook fish fillets for 3-5 minutes per side, or until cooked through.
- While fish is cooking, combine avocado, tomato, red onion, lime juice, and cilantro in a bowl for the salsa.
- For the crema, combine Greek yogurt, lime juice, and cumin in a small bowl.
- Warm tortillas on a griddle or in a skillet.
- Place fish fillets on tortillas, then top with crema and salsa to assemble tacos.

Nutritional Information (per serving):

- Calories: 300-350
- Protein: 30-35 grams
- Carbohydrates: 25-30 grams
- Fat: 15-20 grams

 Keep leftovers in the fridge for up to three days in an airtight container.

To prevent overcooking, reheat the fish and tortillas separately.

Beef Stir-Fry with Brown Rice and Vegetables

Yield: 4 servings **Prep Time:** 20 minutes **Cook Time:** 15-20 minutes

Ingredients:

- 1 pound beef stir-fry strips
- 1 tablespoon olive oil
- 1 onion, chopped
- 1 bell pepper, chopped
- 1 cup broccoli florets
- 1 cup carrots, sliced
- 1 cup cooked brown rice
- 1/4 cup soy sauce
- 1 tablespoon honey
- 1 tablespoon rice vinegar

Instructions:

- In a big skillet set over medium-high heat, warm up the olive oil.
- Cook beef until browned.
- Add onion, bell pepper, broccoli, and carrots. Cook until vegetables are tender-crisp.
- Stir in brown rice, soy sauce, honey, and rice vinegar.
- Cook for 2-3 minutes to combine flavors.

Nutritional Information (per serving):

- Calories: 400-450
- Protein: 30-35 grams
- Carbohydrates: 30-35 grams
- Fat: 15-20 grams

Storage: For up to three days, keep leftovers in the refrigerator in an airtight container.

Warm up again in a skillet over medium heat.

Grilled chicken with a salad of black beans and corn

Yield: 4 servings **Prep Time:** 20 minutes **Cook Time:** 10-15 minutes

Ingredients:

- 1-pound boneless, skinless chicken breasts
- 1 tablespoon olive oil
- Salt and pepper to taste
- One can (15 ounces) of rinsed and drained black beans
- 1 can (15 ounces) corn, drained
- 1 red bell pepper, diced
- 1/4 cup red onion, chopped
- 1/4 cup cilantro, chopped
- 1/4 cup lime juice

Instructions:

- Season chicken breasts with salt and pepper.
- Grill chicken breasts for 10-15 minutes, or until cooked through.
- Let the chicken rest for a few minutes before slicing into strips.
- In a large bowl, combine black beans, corn, red bell pepper, red onion, cilantro, and lime juice.
- Add grilled chicken to the salad and toss to combine.

Nutritional Information (per serving):

Calories: 300-350

Carbohydrates: 30-35 grams

Protein: 30-35 grams

Fat: 10-15 grams

Storage: Keep leftovers in the fridge for up to three days in an airtight container.

Reheating: Reheat gently over low heat to avoid overcooking.

Lentil and Vegetable Chili

Yield: 6 servings **Prep Time:** 30 minutes **Cook Time:** 30-40 minutes

Ingredients:

- 1 tablespoon olive oil
- 1 onion, chopped
- 1 carrot, chopped
- 1 celery stalk, chopped
- Rinse and drain one can (15 ounces) of black beans
- Rinse and drain 1 can (15 ounces) of kidney beans
- 1 can (15 ounces) diced tomatoes
- 1 cup vegetable broth
- 1 teaspoon chili powder
- 1/2 teaspoon cumin
- 1/4 teaspoon garlic powder
- 1/4 teaspoon onion powder
- Salt and pepper to taste

Instructions:

- In a big saucepan, warm up the olive oil over medium heat.
- Add the celery, carrot, and onion. Simmer until tender.
- Add the chili powder, cumin, onion, garlic, and kidney beans along with the chopped tomatoes, vegetable broth, salt, and pepper.
- Bring to a boil, then reduce heat and simmer for 20-30 minutes, or until thickened.

Nutritional Information (per serving):

- Calories: 300-350
- Protein: 20-25 grams
- Carbohydrates: 40-45 grams
- Fat: 10-15 grams

Storage: For up to three days, keep leftovers in the refrigerator in an airtight container.

Reheating: Reheat on the stovetop over medium heat.

Avocado and Spinach Salad with Grilled Chicken

Yield: 4 servings **Prep Time:** 20 minutes **Cook Time:** 15 minutes

Ingredients:

- 1 large avocado, diced
- 1 cup fresh spinach
- 1/2 cup cherry tomatoes, halved
- 1/4 cup red onion, thinly sliced
- 1/4 cup feta cheese, crumbled
- 1/4 cup balsamic vinaigrette dressing
- 1-pound boneless, skinless chicken breasts, grilled and sliced
- Salt and pepper to taste

Instructions:

- In a large bowl, combine the avocado, spinach, cherry tomatoes, red onion, and feta cheese.
- Toss to coat, then drizzle with balsamic vinaigrette dressing.
- Place several pieces of grilled chicken on top and add salt and pepper to taste.

Nutritional Information: (per serving)

- Calories: 400-500
- Protein: 30-35g
- Carbohydrates: 20-25g
- Fat: 25-30g

Storage and Reheating:

- Remaining food can be kept in the refrigerator for up to three days if it is sealed tightly.
- To reheat, gently warm the salad in a pan over low heat or microwave until heated through.

Cauliflower Pizza with Marinara Sauce and Vegetables

Yield: 4 servings **Prep Time:** 30 minutes **Cook Time:** 20-25 minutes

Ingredients:

- 1 head of cauliflower, cut into florets and processed into a pizza crust
- 1/2 cup marinara sauce
- 1/2 cup shredded mozzarella cheese
- 1/2 cup roasted vegetables (e.g., zucchini, bell peppers, mushrooms)
- Fresh basil leaves

Instructions:

- Preheat oven to 400°F (200°C).

- Spread the cauliflower crust on a baking sheet and bake for 10-15 minutes, or until golden brown and crispy.
- Top with marinara sauce, mozzarella cheese, and roasted vegetables.
- Bake for a further ten to fifteen minutes, or until the cheese is bubbling and melted.
- Garnish with fresh basil leaves.

Nutritional Information: (per serving)

- Calories: 300-350
- Protein: 20-25g
- Carbohydrates: 30-35g
- Fat: 15-20g

Storage and Reheating:

- Keep leftovers in the fridge for up to three days in an airtight container.
- To reheat, place leftovers on a baking sheet and bake in a preheated oven at 375°F (190°C) for 10-15 minutes, or until heated through.

Salmon with Roasted Asparagus and Lemon-Dill Sauce

Yield: 4 servings **Prep Time:** 15 minutes **Cook Time:** 15-20 minutes

Ingredients:

- 4 salmon fillets
- 1 bunch of asparagus, trimmed and roasted
- 1/4 cup lemon juice
- 2 tablespoons fresh dill, chopped
- 2 tablespoons olive oil
- Salt and pepper to taste

Instructions:

- Preheat oven to 400°F (200°C).
- Season salmon fillets with salt and pepper.
- Roast asparagus in the oven for 10-15 minutes, or until tender-crisp.
- In a small bowl, whisk together lemon juice, dill, and olive oil.
- Grill or pan-sear salmon fillets until cooked through.
- Serve salmon with roasted asparagus and lemon-dill sauce.

- Calories: 350-400
- Protein: 30-35g
- Carbohydrates: 5-10g
- Fat: 25-30g

Storage and Reheating:

- Keep leftovers in the fridge for up to three days in an airtight container.
- To reheat, gently warm salmon and asparagus in a pan over low heat.

Zucchini Boats Filled with Spinach, Feta, and Tomatoes

Yield: 4 servings **Prep Time:** 20 minutes **Cook Time:** 15-20 minutes

Ingredients:

- 4 large zucchinis
- 1 cup fresh spinach
- 1/2 cup crumbled feta cheese
- 1/2 cup cherry tomatoes, halved
- 2 cloves garlic, minced
- 1/4 cup olive oil
- Salt and pepper to taste

Instructions:

- Preheat oven to 375°F (190°C).
- Cut zucchini lengthwise and scoop out the flesh to create boasts.
- In a bowl, combine spinach, feta cheese, cherry tomatoes, garlic, olive oil, salt, and pepper.
- Fill zucchini boats with the spinach mixture.
- Bake for 15-20 minutes, or until zucchini is tender and filling is heated through.

Nutritional Information: (per serving)

- Calories: 250-300
- Protein: 15-20g
- Carbohydrates: 15-20g
- Fat: 15-20g

Storage and Reheating:

- Keep leftovers in the fridge for up to three days in an airtight container.
- To reheat, place leftovers in a baking dish and bake in a preheated oven at 375°F (190°C) for 10-15 minutes, or until heated through.

Avocado and Tomato Salad with Grilled Shrimp

Yield: 4 servings **Prep Time:** 15 minutes **Cook Time:** 15-20 minutes

Ingredients:

- 1 large avocado, diced
- 1 cup cherry tomatoes, halved
- 1/4 cup red onion, thinly sliced
- 1/4 cup balsamic vinaigrette dressing
- 1-pound large shrimp, peeled and deveined
- Salt and pepper to taste

Instructions:

- In a large bowl, combine the avocado, cherry tomatoes, and red onion.
- Finish by tossing to coat with a balsamic vinaigrette dressing.
- Grill or pan-sear shrimp until cooked through and pink.
- Add grilled shrimp to the salad and season with salt and pepper to taste.

Nutritional Information: (per serving)

- Calories: 350-400
- Protein: 30-35g
- Carbohydrates: 10-15g
- Fat: 25-30g

Storage and Reheating:

- Remaining food can be kept in the refrigerator for up to three days if it is sealed tightly.
- To reheat, gently warm the salad in a pan over low heat or microwave until heated through.

Smoothies

Green Goddess Smoothie

Yield: 2 servings **Prep Time:** 10 minutes **Cook Time:** N/A

Ingredients:

- 1 cup spinach
- 1/2 cucumber, peeled and chopped
- 1/2 avocado
- 1/4 cup Greek yogurt
- 1/4 cup lemon juice
- 1 tablespoon fresh dill
- 1 tablespoon fresh parsley
- 1/2 cup ice

Instructions:

- Smoothly combine all components in a blender after combining them.
- Pour into glasses and enjoy immediately.

Nutritional Information: (per serving)

- Calories: 200-250
- Protein: 10-15g
- Carbohydrates: 20-25g
- Fat: 15-20g

Storage and Reheating:

- Best enjoyed immediately. You may store it in the refrigerator for up to a day by keeping it in an airtight container.

Berry Blast Smoothie

Yield: 2 servings **Prep Time:** 5 minutes **Cook Time:** N/A

Ingredients:

- 1 cup mixed berries (strawberries, raspberries, blueberries)
- 1 banana, sliced
- 1/2 cup Greek yogurt
- 1/2 cup almond milk
- 1 tablespoon honey (optional)
- 1/2 cup ice

Instructions:

- In a blender, combine all ingredients and process until smooth.
- Pour into glasses and enjoy immediately.

Nutritional Information: (per serving)

- Calories: 250-300
- Protein: 10-15g
- Carbohydrates: 30-35g
- Fat: 5-10g

Storage and Reheating:

- Best enjoyed immediately. For up to one day, store in the refrigerator in an airtight container.

Avocado Spinach Smoothie

Yield: 2 servings **Prep Time:** 5 minutes **Cook Time:** N/A

Ingredients:

- 1 avocado
- 1 cup spinach
- 1/2 banana
- 1/2 cup almond milk
- 1/4 cup lemon juice
- 1/2 cup ice

Instructions:

- In a blender, combine all ingredients and process until smooth.
- Pour into glasses and enjoy immediately.

Nutritional Information: (per serving)

- Calories: 250-300
- Protein: 10-15g
- Carbohydrates: 25-30g
- Fat: 20-25g

Storage and Reheating:

- Best enjoyed immediately. For up to one day, store in the refrigerator in an airtight container

Almond Butter Energy Balls

Yield: 12-15 balls **Prep Time:** 15 minutes **Cook Time:** N/A

Ingredients:

- 1 cup almond butter
- 1/4 cup honey
- 1/4 cup rolled oats
- 1/4 cup chocolate chips
- 1/4 cup chia seeds

Instructions:

- In a bowl, combine almond butter, honey, oats, chocolate chips, and chia seeds.
- After thoroughly combining, shape into balls.
- To set, refrigerate for a minimum of half an hour.

Nutritional Information: (per serving)

- Calories: 150-200
- Protein: 5-10g
- Carbohydrates: 15-20g
- Fat: 10-15g

Storage and Reheating:

- Keep refrigerated for up to a week in an airtight container.

Chia Seed Energy Balls

Yield: 12-15 balls **Prep Time:** 15 minutes **Cook Time:** N/A

Ingredients:

- 1/4 cup chia seeds
- 1/4 cup almond milk
- 1/4 cup honey
- 1/4 cup rolled oats
- 1/4 cup chocolate chips

Instructions:

- In a bowl, combine chia seeds, almond milk, honey, oats, and chocolate chips.

- Mix well, then shape into balls.

- Chill for a minimum of half an hour to solidify.

Nutritional Information: (per serving)

- Calories: 100-150
- Protein: 5-10g
- Carbohydrates: 15-20g
- Fat: 5-10g

Storage and Reheating:

- For up to a week, keep in the refrigerator in an airtight container.

Date and Nut Energy Balls

Yield: 12-15 balls **Prep Time:** 15 minutes **Cook Time:** N/A

Ingredients:

- 1 cup pitted dates
- 1/4 cup almond butter
- 1/4 cup walnuts, chopped
- 1/4 cup coconut flakes
- 1/4 teaspoon vanilla extract

Instructions:

- In a food processor, combine dates, almond butter, walnuts, coconut flakes, and vanilla extract.

- Process until well combined and form into balls.

- To set, refrigerate for a minimum of half an hour.

Nutritional Information: (per serving)

- Calories: 150-200
- Protein: 5-10g
- Carbohydrates: 20-25g
- Fat: 10-15g

Storage and Reheating:

- Refrigerate for up to a week after storing in an airtight container.

<u>**Dip and Chips**</u>

Hummus and Vegetable Sticks

Yield: 4 servings **Prep Time:** 15 minutes **Cook Time:** N/A

Ingredients:

- 1 can chickpeas, rinsed and drained
- 1/4 cup tahini
- 1/4 cup lemon juice
- 2 cloves garlic, minced
- 1/4 cup olive oil
- 1/4 cup water
- Salt and pepper to taste
- 1 cup assorted vegetable sticks (carrots, celery, cucumber)

Instructions:

- In a food processor, combine chickpeas, tahini, lemon juice, garlic, olive oil, water, salt, and pepper.
- Process until smooth and creamy.
- Serve with vegetable sticks.

Nutritional Information: (per serving)

- Calories: 200-250
- Protein: 10-15g
- Carbohydrates: 20-25g
- Fat: 15-20g

Storage and Reheating:

- Hummus may be kept in the fridge for up to a week if it is kept in an airtight container.
- Serve with fresh vegetable sticks.

Avocado Dip and Whole Grain Tortilla Chips

Yield: 4 servings **Prep Time:** 15 minutes **Cook Time:** N/A

Ingredients:

- 1 avocado, mashed
- 1/4 cup Greek yogurt
- 1/4 cup lemon juice
- 1 clove garlic, minced
-
- 1/4 cup fresh dill
- Salt and pepper to taste
- 1 bag whole grain tortilla chips

Instructions:

- In a bowl, combine avocado, Greek yogurt, lemon juice, garlic, dill, salt, and pepper.

- Mix until smooth.

- Serve with whole grain tortilla chips.

- Calories: 200-250
- Protein: 10-15g
- Carbohydrates: 20-25g
- Fat: 15-20g

Storage and Reheating:

- Store avocado dip in an airtight container in the refrigerator for up to 3 days.

- Serve with fresh whole grain tortilla chips.

Spinach Artichoke Dip and Pita Bread

Yield: 4 servings **Prep Time:** 15 minutes **Cook Time:** 20-25 minutes

Ingredients:

- Ten ounces of frozen chopped spinach that has been thawed and drained

- 1 (10-ounce) can artichoke hearts, drained and chopped

- 1/2 cup cream cheese, softened

- 1/4 cup Parmesan cheese, grated

- 1/4 cup milk

- 2 cloves garlic, minced

- Salt and pepper to taste

- Pita bread, cut into triangles

Instructions:

- Preheat oven to 375°F (190°C).

- In a large bowl, combine spinach, artichoke hearts, cream cheese, Parmesan cheese, milk, garlic, salt, and pepper.

- Mix until well combined.

- Transfer the blend onto a little baking dish.

- Bake for 20 to 25 minutes, or until bubbling and well cooked.

- Serve with pita bread.

Nutritional Information: (per serving)

- Calories: 250-300
- Protein: 15-20g
- Carbohydrates: 20-25g
- Fat: 15-20g

Storage and Reheating:

- Keep leftovers in the fridge for up to three days in an airtight container.
- To reheat, place leftovers in a baking dish and bake in a preheated oven at 375°F (190°C) for 10-15 minutes, or until heated through.

Trail Mix

Alkaline Trail Mix

Yield: 4 servings **Prep Time:** 15 minutes **Cook Time:** N/A

Ingredients:

- 1 cup almonds
- 1/2 cup cashews
- 1/4 cup pumpkin seeds
- 1/4 cup sunflower seeds
- 1/4 cup dried cranberries
- 1/4 cup raisins
- 1/4 cup dark chocolate chips
- 1 tablespoon honey

Instructions:

- In a large bowl, combine almonds, cashews, pumpkin seeds, sunflower seeds, cranberries, raisins, chocolate chips, and honey.
- Toss to coat.
- Store in an airtight container.

Nutritional Information: (per serving)

- Calories: 250-300
- Protein: 10-15g
- Carbohydrates: 25-30g
- Fat: 15-20g

Storage and Reheating:

- Store in an airtight container in a cool, dry place for up to 2 weeks.

Sweet and Salty Trail Mix

Yield: 4 servings **Prep Time:** 15 minutes **Cook Time:** N/A

Ingredients:

- 1 cup almonds
- 1/2 cup cashews
- 1/4 cup pretzels
- 1/4 cup dried mango
- 1/4 cup dried apricots
- 1/4 cup dark chocolate chips
- 1 tablespoon honey

Instructions:

- In a large bowl, combine almonds, cashews, pretzels, dried mango, dried apricots, chocolate chips, and honey.
- Toss to coat.
- Store in an airtight container.

Nutritional Information: (per serving)

- Calories: 250-300
- Protein: 10-15g
- Carbohydrates: 30-35g
- Fat: 15-20g

Storage and Reheating:

- For up to two weeks, store in an airtight container in a cold, dry location.

Baked Goods

Banana Bread with Almond Flour

Yield: 1 loaf **Prep Time:** 20 minutes **Cook Time:** 45-50 minutes

Ingredients:

- 2 ripe bananas, mashed
- 1/4 cup almond milk
- 1/4 cup maple syrup
- 1/4 cup melted coconut oil
- 1 egg
- 1 teaspoon vanilla extract

- 1 cup almond flour
- 1/2 teaspoon baking powder
- 1/4 teaspoon salt

Instructions:

Instructions:

- Preheat oven to 350°F (175°C).
- Bananas, almond milk, maple syrup, coconut oil, egg, and vanilla extract should all be combined in a big basin.
- Mix the almond flour, baking powder, and salt in another basin.
- Mix until just incorporated, gradually add the dry ingredients to the wet ones.
- Fill a loaf pan with oiled batter.
- When a toothpick put into the center comes out clean, bake for 45 to 50 minutes.

Nutritional Information: (per serving)

- Calories: 250-300
- Protein: 10-15g
- Carbohydrates: 30-35g
- Fat: 15-20g

Storage and Reheating:

- For up to three days, keep in the refrigerator in an airtight container.
- To reheat, slice and toast.

Zucchini Bread with Chia Seeds

Yield: 1 loaf Prep Time: 20 minutes Cook Time: 45-50 minutes

Ingredients:

- 2 cups shredded zucchini
- 1/4 cup almond milk
- 1/4 cup maple syrup
- 1/4 cup melted coconut oil
- 1 egg
- 1 teaspoon vanilla extract
- 1 cup almond flour
- 1/2 cup chia seeds
- 1 teaspoon baking powder
- 1/4 teaspoon salt

Instructions:

- Preheat oven to 350°F (175°C).

- In a large bowl, combine zucchini, almond milk, maple syrup, coconut oil, egg, and vanilla extract.

- In a separate bowl, combine almond flour, chia seeds, baking powder, and salt.

- Mixing until just incorporated, gradually add the dry ingredients to the wet ones.

- Fill a loaf pan with oiled batter.

- When a toothpick put into the center comes out clean, bake for 45 to 50 minutes.

Nutritional Information: (per serving)

- Calories: 250-300
- Protein: 10-15g
- Carbohydrates: 30-35g
- Fat: 15-20g

Storage and Reheating:

- For up to three days, keep in the refrigerator in an airtight container.
- To reheat, slice and toast.

Coconut-Almond Energy Bites

Yield: 15-20 bites Prep Time: 15 minutes Cook Time: N/A

Ingredients:

- 1 cup almond flour
- 1/2 cup unsweetened coconut flakes
- 1/4 cup honey
- 1/4 cup almond butter
- 1/4 cup chocolate chips
- 1/4 teaspoon vanilla extract

Instructions:

- In a large bowl, combine almond flour, coconut flakes, honey, almond butter, chocolate chips, and vanilla extract.
- After thoroughly combining, shape into balls.
- To set, refrigerate for a minimum of half an hour.

Nutritional Information: (per serving)

- Calories: 150-200
- Protein: 5-10g
- Carbohydrates: 20-25g
- Fat: 10-15g

Storage and Reheating:

- For up to a week, keep in the refrigerator in an airtight container.

Fruit and Veggie Snacks

Fruit Salad with a Honey-Lemon Dressing

Yield: 4 servings **Prep Time:** 15 minutes **Cook Time:** N/A

Ingredients:

- 2 cups mixed fruits (e.g., apples, berries, grapes)
- 1/4 cup honey
- 1/4 cup lemon juice
- 2 tablespoons olive oil

Instructions:

- In a large bowl, combine fruits.
- In a small bowl, whisk together honey, lemon juice, and olive oil.
- Pour dressing over fruit salad and toss to coat.

Nutritional Information: (per serving)

- Calories: 150-200
- Protein: 1-2g
- Carbohydrates: 30-35g
- Fat: 5-10g

Storage and Reheating:

- For up to three days, keep in the refrigerator in an airtight container.
- Best served chilled.

Roasted Vegetable Chips

Yield: 4 servings **Prep Time:** 15 minutes **Cook Time:** 20-25 minutes

Ingredients:

- 2 cups mixed vegetables (e.g., sweet potatoes, carrots, zucchini)
- 1 tablespoon olive oil
- 1/2 teaspoon salt
- 1/4 teaspoon paprika

Instructions:

- Preheat oven to 400°F (200°C).
- Cut vegetables into thin slices.
- Toss vegetables with olive oil, salt, and paprika.
- Arrange the veggies on a baking sheet in a single layer.
- Roast for 20-25 minutes, or until crispy.

Nutritional Information: (per serving)

- Calories: 100-150
- Protein: 2-3g
- Carbohydrates: 20-25g
- Fat: 5-10g

Storage and Reheating:

- For up to three days, keep at room temperature in an airtight container.
- Best when consumed raw.

Fruit-Based Desserts

Alkaline Berry Smoothie Bowl

Yield: 2 servings **Prep Time:** 10 minutes **Freezing Time:** N/A (best enjoyed immediately)

Ingredients:

- 1 cup mixed berries (strawberries, raspberries, blueberries)
- 1 banana, sliced
- 1/2 cup Greek yogurt
- 1/4 cup almond milk
- 1 tablespoon honey (optional)
- Toppings: granola, nuts, seeds, fresh fruit

Instructions:

- Combine berries, banana, Greek yogurt, almond milk, and honey in a blender.
- Blend until smooth and creamy.
- Pour into bowls and top with your favorite toppings.

Nutritional Information: (per serving)

- Calories: 250-300
- Protein: 10-15g
- Carbohydrates: 30-35g
- Fat: 5-10g

Storage and Reheating:

- Best enjoyed immediately. For up to one day, store in the refrigerator in an airtight container.

Avocado Chocolate Mousse

Yield: 4 servings **Prep Time:** 15 minutes **Freezing Time:** 2-3 hours

Ingredients:

- 2 ripe avocados
- 1/4 cup maple syrup
- 1/4 cup cocoa powder
- 1/4 cup coconut milk
- 1/4 teaspoon vanilla extract
- Pinch of salt

Instructions:

- In a food processor, combine avocados, maple syrup, cocoa powder, coconut milk, vanilla extract, and salt.
- Process until smooth and creamy.
- Pour into individual serving dishes and refrigerate for at least 2-3 hours, or until set.

Nutritional Information: (per serving)

- Calories: 250-300
- Protein: 5-10g
- Carbohydrates: 25-30g
- Fat: 20-25g

Storage and Reheating:

- Keep leftovers in the fridge for up to three days in an airtight container.
- To serve, let thaw for 15-20 minutes.

Tropical Fruit Chia Seed Pudding

Yield: 4 servings **Prep Time:** 10 minutes **Freezing Time:** N/A (best enjoyed immediately)

Ingredients:

- 1/4 cup chia seeds
- 1 cup almond milk
- 1/4 cup maple syrup
- 1/2 cup chopped mango
- 1/4 cup chopped pineapple
- 1/4 cup chopped papaya

Instructions:

- In a bowl, whisk together chia seeds, almond milk, and maple syrup.
- Let sit for 5-10 minutes, or until thickened.
- Stir in mango, pineapple, and papaya.
- Serve immediately or refrigerate for later.

Nutritional Information: (per serving)

- Calories: 150-200
- Protein: 5-10g
- Carbohydrates: 20-25g
- Fat: 10-15g

Storage and Reheating:

- Remaining food can be kept in the refrigerator for up to three days if it is sealed tightly.
- To serve, let thaw for 15-20 minutes.

Lemon Blueberry Sorbet

Yield: 4 servings **Prep Time:** 15 minutes **Freezing Time:** 2-3 hours

Ingredients:

- 2 cups fresh blueberries
- 1/2 cup lemon juice
- 1/4 cup maple syrup
- 1/4 cup water

Instructions:

- In a blender, combine blueberries, lemon juice, maple syrup, and water.
- Blend until smooth.
- Pour into a freezer-safe container and freeze for 2-3 hours, or until firm.
- Break up the sorbet with a fork before serving.

Nutritional Information: (per serving)

- Calories: 150-200
- Protein: 1-2g
- Carbohydrates: 30-35g
- Fat: 1-2g

Storage and Reheating:

- Remaining food can be kept in the freezer for up to two months if it is sealed tightly.
- Let thaw for 15-20 minutes before serving.

Mango Avocado Ice Cream

Yield: 4 servings **Prep Time:** 15 minutes **Freezing Time:** 2-3 hours

Ingredients:

- 1 ripe avocado
- 1 cup frozen mango chunks
- 1/4 cup maple syrup
- 1/4 cup coconut milk
- Pinch of salt

Instructions:

- In a food processor, combine avocado, mango, maple syrup, coconut milk, and salt.
- Process until smooth and creamy.
- Pour into a freezer-safe container and freeze for 2-3 hours, or until firm.
- Break up the ice cream with a fork before serving.

Nutritional Information: (per serving)

- Calories: 250-300
- Protein: 5-10g
- Carbohydrates: 30-35g
- Fat: 20-25g

- Remaining food can be kept in the freezer for up to two months if it is sealed tightly.
- Let thaw for 15-20 minutes before serving.

Alkaline Apple Crisp

Yield: 4 servings **Prep Time:** 20 minutes **Cook Time:** 30-35 minutes

Ingredients:

- 4 apples, peeled, cored, and sliced
- 1/4 cup maple syrup
- 1/4 cup lemon juice
- 1/4 cup almond flour
- 1/4 cup rolled oats
- 1/4 cup coconut sugar
- 1/4 cup chopped walnuts

Instructions:

- Preheat oven to 375°F (190°C).
- In a bowl, combine apples, maple syrup, and lemon juice.
- Pour apple mixture into a baking dish.
- In a separate bowl, combine almond flour, rolled oats, coconut sugar, and walnuts.
- Crumble the oat mixture over the apple mixture.
- Bake for thirty to thirty-five minutes, or until the apples are soft and the topping is browned.

Nutritional Information: (per serving)

- Calories: 250-300
- Protein: 5-10g
- Carbohydrates: 30-35g
- Fat: 15-20g

Storage and Reheating:

- Remaining food can be kept in the refrigerator for up to three days if it is sealed tightly.
- To reheat, place leftovers in a baking dish and bake in a preheated oven at 375°F (190°C) for 10-15 minutes, or until heated through.

Raspberry Lemon Tart

Yield: 8 servings **Prep Time:** 30 minutes **Cook Time:** 30-35 minutes

Ingredients:

- 1 graham cracker crust
- 1 cup raspberries
- 1/4 cup lemon juice
- 1/4 cup maple syrup
- 1/4 cup almond flour
- 1/4 cup coconut sugar

Instructions:

- Preheat oven to 375°F (190°C).
- In a bowl, combine raspberries, lemon juice, maple syrup, almond flour, and coconut sugar.
- Pour filling into prepared graham cracker crust.
- Bake for 30-35 minutes, or until set.
- Let cool completely before serving.

Nutritional Information: (per serving)

- Calories: 250-300
- Protein: 5-10g
- Carbohydrates: 30-35g
- Fat: 15-20g

Storage and Reheating:

- Refrigerate leftovers in an airtight jar for up to three days.
- Allow to defrost for 15-20 minutes before serving.

Nut-Based Desserts

Almond Butter and Banana Bites

Yield: 12-15 bites **Prep Time:** 15 minutes **Freezing Time:** N/A (best enjoyed fresh)

Ingredients:

- 1/2 cup almond butter
- 1/4 cup honey
- 1/4 cup rolled oats
- 1/4 cup chocolate chips

- 1 banana, sliced

Instructions:

- In a bowl, combine almond butter, honey, oats, and chocolate chips.
- Mix until well combined.
- Roll into bite-sized balls and coat with sliced banana.

Nutritional Information: (per serving)

- Calories: 150-200
- Protein: 5-10g
- Carbohydrates: 20-25g
- Fat: 10-15g

Storage and Reheating:

- Best enjoyed fresh. If storing, keep in an airtight container in the refrigerator for up to 1 week.

Cashew Cream Tartlets

Yield: 12 tartlets **Prep Time:** 30 minutes **Freezing Time:** N/A (best enjoyed fresh)

Ingredients:

- 1 cup cashews, soaked overnight
- 1/4 cup maple syrup
- 1/4 cup lemon juice
- 1/4 cup coconut oil, melted
- 1 teaspoon vanilla extract
- 12 mini tart shells
- Fresh berries for topping

Instructions:

- Drain and rinse-soaked cashews.
- In a food processor, combine cashews, maple syrup, lemon juice, coconut oil, and vanilla extract.
- Process until smooth and creamy.
- Fill tart shells with cashew cream and top with fresh berries.

Nutritional Information: (per serving)

- Calories: 200-250
- Protein: 5-10g
- Carbohydrates: 20-25g
- Fat: 15-20g

Storage and Reheating:

- Best enjoyed fresh. If storing, keep in an airtight container in the refrigerator for up to 1 week.

Walnut and Date Energy Balls

Yield: 12-15 balls **Prep Time:** 15 minutes **Freezing Time:** N/A (best enjoyed fresh)

Ingredients:

- 1 cup pitted dates
- 1/4 cup walnuts, chopped
- 1/4 cup almond butter
- 1/4 cup coconut flakes
- 1/4 teaspoon vanilla extract

Instructions:

- In a food processor, combine dates, walnuts, almond butter, coconut flakes, and vanilla extract.
- Process until well combined and form into balls.

Nutritional Information: (per serving)

- Calories: 150-200
- Protein: 5-10g
- Carbohydrates: 20-25g
- Fat: 10-15g

Storage and Reheating:

- Refrigerate in an airtight container for up to a week.

Chia Seed Almond Pudding

Yield: 4 servings **Prep Time:** 5 minutes **Freezing Time:** N/A (best enjoyed fresh)

Ingredients:

- 1/4 cup chia seeds
- 1 cup almond milk
- 1/4 cup honey
- 1/4 teaspoon vanilla extract
- Toppings: fresh berries, nuts, granola

Instructions:

- In a mixing dish, add chia seeds, almond milk, honey, and vanilla essence.
- Stir until well blended.
- Cover and chill for at least 2 hours, preferably overnight, to allow the chia seeds to grow.
- Serve with your desired toppings.

Nutritional Information: (per serving)

- Calories: 150-200
- Protein: 5-10g
- Carbohydrates: 20-25g
- Fat: 10-15g

Storage and Reheating:

- Refrigerate in an airtight container for up to three days.

Pumpkin Seed Brittle

Yield: 1 large sheet Prep Time: 15 minutes Cook Time: 15-20 minutes

Ingredients:

- 1 cup pumpkin seeds
- 1/4 cup maple syrup
- 1/4 cup honey
- 1/4 teaspoon salt

Instructions:

- Preheat oven to 350°F (175°C).
- Line a baking sheet with parchment paper.
- In a small saucepan, combine pumpkin seeds, maple syrup, honey, and salt.
- Bring to a boil, then reduce heat and simmer for 5-7 minutes, stirring frequently, until the mixture thickens.
- Pour the mixture onto the baking sheet and distribute evenly.
- Let cool completely before breaking into pieces.

Nutritional Information: (per serving)

- Calories: 200-250
- Protein: 5-10g
- Carbohydrates: 20-25g
- Fat: 15-20g

Storage and Reheating:

Refrigerate in an airtight container for up to one week.

Grain-Free Desserts

Coconut Almond Flour Cookies

Yield: 24 cookies Prep Time: 30 minutes Freezing Time: 1 hour

Ingredients:

- 1 cup almond flour
- 1/2 cup coconut flour
- 1/2 cup coconut oil, melted
- 1/4 cup maple syrup
- 1 large egg
- 1 teaspoon vanilla extract
- 1/4 cup chocolate chips

Instructions:

- Preheat oven to 350°F (175°C).
- In a large bowl, whisk together almond flour, coconut flour, melted coconut oil, maple syrup, egg, and vanilla extract.
- Stir in chocolate chips.
- Drop onto a baking sheet covered with parchment paper by rounded teaspoons.
- Bake for 10-12 minutes, or until golden brown.

- Let cool on baking sheet for a few minutes before transferring to a wire rack to cool completely.

- Calories: 150-200
- Protein: 5-7g
- Carbohydrates: 15-20g
- Fat: 10-15g

Storage and Reheating:

- Refrigerate cookies in an airtight container for up to a week.
- Place the cookies in a freezer-safe container or bag and freeze for up to three months.
- To reheat, let cookies thaw at room temperature or microwave for a few seconds.

Almond Flour Chocolate Cake

Yield: 10-12 servings Prep Time: 30 minutes Cook Time: 30-35 minutes

Ingredients:

- 1 cup almond flour
- 1/2 cup coconut flour
- 1/2 cup cocoa powder
- 1/2 cup maple syrup
- 1/4 cup melted coconut oil
- 1/4 cup almond milk
- 2 large eggs
- 1 teaspoon vanilla extract
- 1 teaspoon baking powder
- 1/2 teaspoon baking soda
- 1/4 teaspoon salt
- 1/2 cup chocolate chips

Instructions:

- Preheat oven to 350°F (175°C). Grease and flour a nine-inch circular cake pan.
- In a big mixing bowl, combine almond flour, coconut flour, cocoa powder, maple syrup, coconut oil, almond milk, eggs, vanilla extract, baking powder, baking soda, and salt.
- Add chocolate chips.
- Pour the batter into the pan and bake for 30-35 minutes, or until a toothpick inserted in the middle comes out clean.
- Allow to cool in pan for 10 minutes before transferring to a wire rack to cool fully.

Nutritional Information: (per serving)

- Calories: 300-350
- Protein: 10-15g
- Carbohydrates: 30-35g
- Fat: 20-25g

Storage and Reheating:

- Refrigerate cake in an airtight container for up to three days.

- To freeze, let cake cool completely, wrap in plastic wrap, and then aluminum foil. Freeze for up to 3 months.
- To thaw, let cake thaw overnight in the refrigerator.
- To reheat, place cake in a preheated oven at 350°F (175°C) for 10-15 minutes.

Chia Seed Raspberry Jam Bars

Yield: 12 bars **Prep Time:** 20 minutes **Cook Time:** 20-25 minutes

Ingredients:

- 1 cup chia seeds
- 1/2 cup almond milk
- 1/4 cup maple syrup
- 1/4 cup coconut oil, melted
- 1 teaspoon vanilla extract
- 1 cup raspberry jam
- 1/4 cup almond flour

Instructions:

- In a bowl, combine chia seeds, almond milk, maple syrup, coconut oil, and vanilla extract.
- Let sit for 10 minutes, or until thickened.
- Press chia seed mixture into the bottom of a 9x9 inch baking pan.
- Spread raspberry jam evenly over the chia seed layer.
- Sprinkle almond flour over the top.
- Bake for 20-25 minutes, or until golden brown.
- Let cool completely before cutting into bars.

Nutritional Information: (per bar)

- Calories: 150-200
- Protein: 5-10g
- Carbohydrates: 20-25g
- Fat: 10-15g

Storage and Reheating:

- Refrigerate bars in an airtight jar for up to three days.
- To freeze, cut bars into individual pieces and place in a freezer-safe container. Freeze for up to 3 months.
- To reheat, let bars thaw at room temperature.

21-Day Low-Sugar Meal Plan

Purpose: To manage blood sugar levels, particularly beneficial for individuals with insulin resistance, diabetes, or those looking to reduce sugar intake.

Key Features:

- Focuses on low glycemic index foods (berries, nuts, leafy greens) to maintain stable blood sugar levels.
- Incorporates plenty of fiber-rich vegetables and whole grains to slow the absorption of sugar.
- Inclusion of healthy fats (avocado, nuts) and lean proteins (legumes) to balance meals.
- Use of natural sweeteners like stevia or monk fruit instead of refined sugars.
- Avoidance of refined carbohydrates, sugary drinks, and processed foods.

Day 1

- **Breakfast:** Green Goddess Smoothie (2 servings)
- **Lunch:** Kale and Quinoa Salad (1 serving)
- **Dinner:** Grilled Salmon with Roasted Vegetables (1 serving)
- **Snack:** Almond Butter and Berry Oatmeal (1 serving)

Day 2

- **Breakfast:** Berry Blast Smoothie (2 servings)
- **Lunch:** Avocado and Spinach Salad (1 serving)
- **Dinner:** Lentil and Vegetable Curry (1 serving)
- **Snack:** Chia Seed Energy Balls (2 servings)

Day 3

- **Breakfast:** Avocado Almond Smoothie (2 servings)
- **Lunch:** Roasted Vegetable Salad (1 serving)
- **Dinner:** Grilled Chicken Breast with Lemon-Herb Marinade and Steamed Broccoli (1 serving)
- **Snack:** Hummus and Vegetable Sticks (2 servings)

Day 4

- **Breakfast:** Tropical Paradise Smoothie (2 servings)
- **Lunch:** Spinach and Feta Wrap (1 serving)
- **Dinner:** Tofu Scramble with Spinach and Tomatoes (1 serving)
- **Snack:** Spinach Artichoke Dip and Pita Bread (2 servings)

Day 5

- **Breakfast:** Spinach and Cucumber Smoothie (2 servings)
- **Lunch:** Buddha Bowl (1 serving)
- **Dinner:** Shrimp Scampi with Zucchini Noodles (1 serving)
- **Snack:** Date and Nut Energy Balls (2 servings)

Day 6

- **Breakfast:** Oatmeal Variations (1 serving)
- **Lunch:** Power Bowl (1 serving)
- **Dinner:** Black Bean and Corn Salad with Grilled Chicken (1 serving)
- **Snack:** Fruit Salad with a Honey-Lemon Dressing (1 serving)

Day 7

- **Breakfast:** Almond Butter and Berry Oatmeal (1 serving)
- **Lunch:** Grain Bowl (1 serving)
- **Dinner:** Roasted Vegetable Medley with Quinoa (1 serving)
- **Snack:** Alkaline Trail Mix (1 serving)

Day 8

- **Breakfast:** Chia Seed and Coconut Oatmeal (1 serving)
- **Lunch:** Salad Bowl (1 serving)
- **Dinner:** Lentil and Vegetable Chili (1 serving)
- **Snack:** Coconut Almond Flour Cookies (2 cookies)

Day 9

- **Breakfast:** Pumpkin Spice Oatmeal (1 serving)
- **Lunch:** Smoothie Bowl (1 serving)
- **Dinner:** Avocado and Tomato Salad with Grilled Shrimp (1 serving)
- **Snack:** Almond Butter and Banana Bites (2 servings)

Day 10

- **Breakfast:** Scrambled Eggs with Spinach and Tomatoes (1 serving)

- **Lunch:** Hummus and Veggie Wrap (1 serving)
- **Dinner:** Baked Chicken Breast with Roasted Brussels Sprouts (1 serving)
- **Snack:** Cashew Cream Tartlets (2 servings)

Day 11

- **Breakfast:** Avocado Toast with a Poached Egg (1 serving)
- **Lunch:** Spinach and Feta Wrap (1 serving)
- **Dinner:** Fish Tacos with Avocado Salsa and Lime Crema (1 serving)
- **Snack:** Walnut and Date Energy Balls (2 servings)

Day 12

- **Breakfast:** Hard-Boiled Eggs with Alkaline-Forming Salad (1 serving)
- **Lunch:** Grain Bowl (1 serving)
- **Dinner:** Roasted Beet Salad with Goat Cheese and Walnuts (1 serving)
- **Snack:** Chia Seed Raspberry Jam Bars (2 bars)

Day 13

- **Breakfast:** Quinoa Porridge with Berries and Nuts (1 serving)
- **Lunch:** Buddha Bowl (1 serving)
- **Dinner:** Green Bean and Potato Casserole (1 serving)
- **Snack:** Alkaline Berry Smoothie Bowl (2 servings)

Day 14

- **Breakfast:** Buckwheat Pancakes with Fruit (1 serving)
- **Lunch:** Salad Bowl (1 serving)
- **Dinner:** Grilled Zucchini and Squash with Avocado Pesto (1 serving)
- **Snack:** Tropical Fruit Chia Seed Pudding (1 serving)

Day 15

- **Breakfast:** Hemp Seed Pudding with Coconut Milk (1 serving)
- **Lunch:** Lentil and Cucumber Salad (1 serving)
- **Dinner:** Cauliflower Steak with Lemon-Herb Sauce (1 serving)
- **Snack:** Avocado Chocolate Mousse (1 serving)

Day 16

- **Breakfast:** Alkaline-Forming Granola with Yogurt (1 serving)
- **Lunch:** Roasted Vegetable Salad (1 serving)
- **Dinner:** Asparagus and Salmon Salad with Lemon-Dill Dressing (1 serving)

- **Snack:** Mango Avocado Ice Cream (1 serving)

Day 17

- **Breakfast:** Scrambled Eggs with Spinach and Tomatoes (1 serving)
- **Lunch:** Spinach and Feta Wrap (1 serving)
- **Dinner:** Stir-Fried Vegetables with Tofu (1 serving)
- **Snack:** Pumpkin Seed Brittle (1 serving)

Day 18

- **Breakfast:** Avocado Toast with a Poached Egg (1 serving)
- **Lunch:** Grain Bowl (1 serving)
- **Dinner:** Roasted Vegetable Soup with Coconut Milk (1 serving)
- **Snack:** Almond Butter and Banana Bites (2 servings)

Day 19

- **Breakfast:** Hard-Boiled Eggs with Alkaline-Forming Salad (1 serving)
- **Lunch:** Buddha Bowl (1 serving)
- **Dinner:** Lentil and Vegetable Curry (1 serving)
- **Snack:** Tropical Fruit Chia Seed Pudding (1 serving)

Day 20

- **Breakfast:** Quinoa Porridge with Berries and Nuts (1 serving)
- **Lunch:** Salad Bowl (1 serving)
- **Dinner:** Grilled Vegetable Medley with Quinoa (1 serving)
- **Snack:** Alkaline Berry Smoothie Bowl (2 servings)

Day 21

- **Breakfast:** Buckwheat Pancakes with Fruit (1 serving)
- **Lunch:** Lentil and Cucumber Salad (1 serving)
- **Dinner:** Roasted Beet Salad with Goat Cheese and Walnuts (1 serving)
- **Snack:** Coconut Almond Flour Cookies (2 cookies)

21-Day Hormone-Balancing Meal Plan

Purpose: To support hormonal balance, especially for individuals dealing with hormonal imbalances, menopause, or menstrual irregularities.

Key Features:

- Rich in healthy fats (avocado, olive oil, nuts)
- Inclusion of cruciferous vegetables (broccoli, cauliflower, kale)
- Emphasis on fiber-rich foods
- Incorporation of phytoestrogen-rich foods (flaxseeds, soy in moderation)
- Avoidance of caffeine, alcohol, and processed foods

Day 1

- **Breakfast:** Almond Butter and Berry Oatmeal (1 serving)
- **Lunch:** Kale and Quinoa Salad (1 serving)
- **Snack:** Almond Butter and Banana Bites (2)
- **Dinner:** Grilled Salmon with Roasted Vegetables (1 serving)
- **Snack:** Green Goddess Smoothie (1 serving)

Day 2

- **Breakfast:** Scrambled Eggs with Spinach and Tomatoes (1 serving)
- **Lunch:** Lentil and Cucumber Salad (1 serving)
- **Snack:** Cashew Cream Tartlets (2)
- **Dinner:** Grilled Chicken Breast with Lemon-Herb Marinade and Steamed Broccoli (1 serving)
- **Snack:** Tropical Paradise Smoothie (1 serving)

Day 3

- **Breakfast:** Spinach and Avocado Oatmeal (1 serving)
- **Lunch:** Buddha Bowl (1 serving)
- **Snack:** Walnut and Date Energy Balls (2)
- **Dinner:** Roasted Vegetable Medley with Quinoa (1 serving)
- **Snack:** Berry Blast Smoothie (1 serving)

Day 4

- **Breakfast:** Pumpkin Spice Oatmeal (1 serving)

- **Lunch:** Hummus and Veggie Wrap (1 serving)
- **Snack:** Chia Seed Almond Pudding (1 serving)
- **Dinner:** Tofu Scramble with Spinach and Tomatoes (1 serving)
- **Snack:** Avocado Spinach Smoothie (1 serving)

Day 5

- **Breakfast:** Chia Seed Pudding with Egg Whites (1 serving)
- **Lunch:** Buddha Bowl (1 serving)
- **Snack:** Pumpkin Seed Brittle (1 serving)
- **Dinner:** Beef Stir-Fry with Brown Rice and Vegetables (1 serving)
- **Snack:** Green Goddess Smoothie (1 serving)

Day 6

Breakfast: Almond Butter and Berry Oatmeal (1 serving)

Lunch: Hummus and Veggie Wrap (1 serving)

Snack: Coconut Almond Flour Cookies (2)

Dinner: Lentil and Vegetable Chili (1 serving)

Snack: Berry Blast Smoothie (1 serving)

Day 7

- **Breakfast:** Tropical Fruit Oatmeal (1 serving)
- **Lunch:** Power Bowl (1 serving)
- **Snack:** Almond Butter and Banana Bites (2)
- **Dinner:** Grilled Salmon with Roasted Vegetables (1 serving)
- **Snack:** Avocado Spinach Smoothie (1 serving)

Day 8

- **Breakfast:** Berry Blast Smoothie (1 serving)
- **Lunch:** Kale and Quinoa Salad (1 serving)
- **Snack:** Cashew Cream Tartlets (2)
- **Dinner:** Roasted Vegetable Soup with Coconut Milk (1 serving)
- **Snack:** Tropical Paradise Smoothie (1 serving)

Day 9

- **Breakfast:** Hard-Boiled Eggs with Alkaline-Forming Salad (1 serving)
- **Lunch:** Grain Bowl (1 serving)
- **Snack:** Walnut and Date Energy Balls (2)
- **Dinner:** Chicken Scampi with Zucchini Noodles (1 serving)

- Snack: Berry Blast Smoothie (1 serving)

Day 10

- Breakfast: Tropical Paradise Smoothie (1 serving)
- Lunch: Spinach and Feta Wrap (1 serving)
- Snack: Chia Seed Almond Pudding (1 serving)
- Dinner: Baked Chicken Breast with Roasted Brussels Sprouts (1 serving)
- Snack: Green Goddess Smoothie (1 serving)

Day 11

- Breakfast: Pumpkin Spice Oatmeal (1 serving)
- Lunch: Hummus and Veggie Wrap (1 serving)
- Snack: Coconut Almond Flour Cookies (2)
- Dinner: Fish Tacos with Avocado Salsa and Lime Crema (1 serving)
- Snack: Tropical Paradise Smoothie (1 serving)

Day 12

- Breakfast: Chia Seed Pudding with Egg Whites (1 serving)
- Lunch: Buddha Bowl (1 serving)
- Snack: Pumpkin Seed Brittle (1 serving)

- Dinner: Beef Stir-Fry with Brown Rice and Vegetables (1 serving)
- Snack: Avocado Spinach Smoothie (1 serving)

Day 13

- Breakfast: Almond Butter and Berry Oatmeal (1 serving)
- Lunch: Hummus and Veggie Wrap (1 serving)
- Snack: Coconut Almond Flour Cookies (2)
- Dinner: Lentil and Vegetable Chili (1 serving)
- Snack: Berry Blast Smoothie (1 serving)

Day 14

- Breakfast: Tropical Fruit Oatmeal (1 serving)
- Lunch: Power Bowl (1 serving)
- Snack: Almond Butter and Banana Bites (2)
- Dinner: Grilled Salmon with Roasted Vegetables (1 serving)
- Snack: Avocado Spinach Smoothie (1 serving)

Day 15

- Breakfast: Green Goddess Smoothie (1 serving)

- **Lunch:** Kale and Quinoa Salad (1 serving)
- **Snack:** Cashew Cream Tartlets (2)
- **Dinner:** Roasted Vegetable Medley with Quinoa (1 serving)
- **Snack:** Tropical Paradise Smoothie (1 serving)

Day 16

- **Breakfast:** Scrambled Eggs with Spinach and Tomatoes (1 serving)
- **Lunch:** Lentil and Cucumber Salad (1 serving)
- **Snack:** Walnut and Date Energy Balls (2)
- **Dinner:** Grilled Chicken Breast with Lemon-Herb Marinade and Steamed Broccoli (1 serving)
- **Snack:** Berry Blast Smoothie (1 serving)

Day 17

- **Breakfast:** Spinach and Avocado Oatmeal (1 serving)
- **Lunch:** Buddha Bowl (1 serving)
- **Snack:** Chia Seed Almond Pudding (1 serving)
- **Dinner:** Tofu Scramble with Spinach and Tomatoes (1 serving)
- **Snack:** Green Goddess Smoothie (1 serving)

Day 18

- **Breakfast:** Pumpkin Spice Oatmeal (1 serving)
- **Lunch:** Hummus and Veggie Wrap (1 serving)
- **Snack:** Coconut Almond Flour Cookies (2)
- **Dinner:** Fish Tacos with Avocado Salsa and Lime Crema (1 serving)
- **Snack:** Tropical Paradise Smoothie (1 serving)

Day 19

- **Breakfast:** Chia Seed Pudding with Egg Whites (1 serving)
- **Lunch:** Buddha Bowl (1 serving)
- **Snack:** Pumpkin Seed Brittle (1 serving)
- **Dinner:** Beef Stir-Fry with Brown Rice and Vegetables (1 serving)
- **Snack:** Avocado Spinach Smoothie (1 serving)

Day 20

- **Breakfast:** Almond Butter and Berry Oatmeal (1 serving)
- **Lunch:** Hummus and Veggie Wrap (1 serving)
- **Snack:** Coconut Almond Flour Cookies (2)

- **Dinner:** Lentil and Vegetable Chili (1 serving)
- **Snack:** Berry Blast Smoothie (1 serving)

Day 21

Breakfast: Tropical Fruit Oatmeal (1 serving)

Remember to:

- Drink plenty of water throughout the day.
- Avoid processed foods, caffeine, and alcohol.
- Listen to your body and adjust as needed.

21-Day Alkaline Weight Loss Meal Plan

Day 1:

- **Breakfast:** Green Goddess Smoothie (1 large glass)
- **Snack:** Almond Butter Energy Balls (2 balls)
- **Lunch:** Kale and Quinoa Salad (1 bowl)
- **Snack:** Hummus and Vegetable Sticks (1 cup vegetables with 2 tbsp hummus)
- **Dinner:** Grilled Salmon with Roasted Vegetables (1 salmon fillet with 1 cup mixed roasted vegetables)

Day 2:

- **Breakfast:** Almond Butter and Berry Oatmeal (1 bowl)
- **Snack:** Fruit Salad with Honey-Lemon Dressing (1 cup)

Lunch: Power Bowl (1 serving)

Snack: Almond Butter and Banana Bites (2)

Dinner: Grilled Salmon with Roasted Vegetables (1 serving)

Snack: Avocado Spinach Smoothie (1 serving)

- **Lunch:** Spinach and Feta Wrap (1 wrap)
- **Snack:** Alkaline Trail Mix (1/4 cup)
- **Dinner:** Cauliflower Steak with Lemon-Herb Sauce (1 cauliflower steak with 2 tbsp sauce)

Day 3:

- **Breakfast:** Avocado Almond Smoothie (1 large glass)
- **Snack:** Banana Bread with Almond Flour (1 slice)
- **Lunch:** Lentil and Cucumber Salad (1 bowl)
- **Snack:** Date and Nut Energy Balls (2 balls)
- **Dinner:** Stir-Fried Vegetables with Tofu (1 bowl)

Day 4:

- **Breakfast:** Chia Seed and Coconut Oatmeal (1 bowl)
- **Snack:** Roasted Vegetable Chips (1 cup)
- **Lunch:** Hummus and Veggie Wrap (1 wrap)
- **Snack:** Almond Butter Energy Balls (2 balls)
- **Dinner:** Roasted Beet Salad with Goat Cheese and Walnuts (1 bowl)

Day 5:

- **Breakfast:** Berry Blast Smoothie (1 large glass)
- **Snack:** Chia Seed Raspberry Jam Bars (2 bars)
- **Lunch:** Lentil Soup (1 bowl)
- **Snack:** Sweet and Salty Trail Mix (1/4 cup)
- **Dinner:** Grilled Zucchini and Squash with Avocado Pesto (1 plate)

Day 6:

- **Breakfast:** Tropical Paradise Smoothie (1 large glass)
- **Snack:** Avocado Dip and Whole Grain Tortilla Chips (1/2 cup dip with 10 chips)
- **Lunch:** Roasted Vegetable Salad (1 bowl)

- **Snack:** Coconut-Almond Energy Bites (2 bites)
- **Dinner:** Tofu Scramble with Spinach and Tomatoes (1 plate)

Day 7:

- **Breakfast:** Pumpkin Spice Oatmeal (1 bowl)
- **Snack:** Cashew Cream Tartlets (2 tartlets)
- **Lunch:** Buddha Bowl (1 bowl)
- **Snack:** Hummus and Vegetable Sticks (1 cup vegetables with 2 tbsp hummus)
- **Dinner:** Grilled Salmon with Lemon-Dill Sauce and Roasted Asparagus (1 salmon fillet with 1 cup asparagus)

Day 8:

- **Breakfast:** Spinach and Cucumber Smoothie (1 large glass)
- **Snack:** Coconut Almond Flour Cookies (2 cookies)
- **Lunch:** Beetroot and Goat Cheese Salad (1 bowl)
- **Snack:** Pumpkin Seed Brittle (2 pieces)
- **Dinner:** Lentil and Vegetable Curry (1 bowl)

Day 9:

- **Breakfast:** Scrambled Eggs with Spinach and Tomatoes (2 eggs with 1 cup vegetables)
- **Snack:** Raspberry Lemon Tart (1 tart)
- **Lunch:** Power Bowl (1 bowl)
- **Snack:** Avocado Spinach Smoothie (1 large glass)
- **Dinner:** Turkey Burgers with Avocado Mayo and Sweet Potato Fries (1 burger with 1/2 cup fries)

Day 10:

- **Breakfast:** Spinach and Avocado Oatmeal (1 bowl)
- **Snack:** Fruit Salad with Honey-Lemon Dressing (1 cup)
- **Lunch:** Grilled Vegetable Wrap (1 wrap)
- **Snack:** Date and Nut Energy Balls (2 balls)
- **Dinner:** Lentil and Vegetable Chili (1 bowl)

Day 11:

- **Breakfast:** Oatmeal with Tropical Fruit (1 bowl)
- **Snack:** Coconut-Almond Energy Bites (2 bites)
- **Lunch:** Grain Bowl (1 bowl)

- **Snack:** Hummus and Vegetable Sticks (1 cup vegetables with 2 tbsp hummus)
- **Dinner:** Shrimp Scampi with Zucchini Noodles (1 plate)

Day 12:

- **Breakfast:** Avocado Toast with Lemon and Herbs (1 slice)
- **Snack:** Banana Bread with Almond Flour (1 slice)
- **Lunch:** Tomato Soup (1 bowl)
- **Snack:** Alkaline Trail Mix (1/4 cup)
- **Dinner:** Cauliflower Pizza with Marinara Sauce and Vegetables (2 slices)

Day 13:

- **Breakfast:** Chia Seed Pudding with Egg Whites (1 bowl)
- **Snack:** Energy Balls (Almond Butter) (2 balls)
- **Lunch:** Smoothie Bowl (1 bowl)
- **Snack:** Zucchini Bread with Chia Seeds (1 slice)
- **Dinner:** Asparagus and Salmon Salad with Lemon-Dill Dressing (1 plate)

Day 14:

- **Breakfast:** Omelet with Vegetables and Herbs (1 omelet with 1 cup mixed vegetables)

- **Snack:** Coconut Almond Flour Cookies (2 cookies)
- **Lunch:** Lentil Soup (1 bowl)
- **Snack:** Sweet and Salty Trail Mix (1/4 cup)
- **Dinner:** Grilled Chicken with Roasted Brussels Sprouts (1 chicken breast with 1 cup sprouts)

Day 15:

- **Breakfast:** Green Goddess Smoothie (1 large glass)
- **Snack:** Avocado Chocolate Mousse (1/2 cup)
- **Lunch:** Buddha Bowl (1 bowl)
- **Snack:** Fruit Salad with Honey-Lemon Dressing (1 cup)
- **Dinner:** Fish Tacos with Avocado Salsa and Lime Crema (2 tacos)

Day 16:

- **Breakfast:** Berry Blast Smoothie (1 large glass)
- **Snack:** Chia Seed Energy Balls (2 balls)
- **Lunch:** Avocado and Spinach Salad (1 bowl)
- **Snack:** Roasted Vegetable Chips (1 cup)
- **Dinner:** Roasted Vegetable Soup with Coconut Milk (1 bowl)

Day 17:

- **Breakfast:** Almond Butter and Berry Oatmeal (1 bowl)
- **Snack:** Chia Seed Almond Pudding (1 bowl)
- **Lunch:** Hummus and Veggie Wrap (1 wrap)
- **Snack:** Coconut-Almond Energy Bites (2 bites)
- **Dinner:** Beef Stir-Fry with Brown Rice and Vegetables (1 plate)

Day 18:

- **Breakfast:** Tropical Paradise Smoothie (1 large glass)
- **Snack:** Pumpkin Seed Brittle (2 pieces)
- **Lunch:** Salad Bowl (1 bowl)
- **Snack:** Energy Balls (Chia Seed) (2 balls)
- **Dinner:** Black Bean and Corn Salad with Grilled Chicken (1 bowl)

Day 19:

- **Breakfast:** Spinach and Cucumber Smoothie (1 large glass)
- **Snack:** Zucchini Bread with Chia Seeds (1 slice)
- **Lunch:** Lentil and Quinoa Wrap (1 wrap)
- **Snack:** Alkaline Trail Mix (1/4 cup)

- **Dinner:** Grilled Salmon with Roasted Vegetables (1 salmon fillet with 1 cup mixed roasted vegetables)

Day 20:

- **Breakfast:** Pumpkin Spice Oatmeal (1 bowl)
- **Snack:** Avocado Spinach Smoothie (1 large glass)
- **Lunch:** Roasted Vegetable Salad (1 bowl)
- **Snack:** Coconut-Almond Energy Bites (2 bites)

- **Dinner:** Zucchini Boats Filled with Spinach, Feta, and Tomatoes (2 boats)

Day 21:

- **Breakfast:** Avocado Toast with a Poached Egg (1 slice toast with 1 egg)
- **Snack:** Fruit Salad with Honey-Lemon Dressing (1 cup)
- **Lunch:** Vegetable Soup (1 bowl)
- **Snack:** Energy Balls (Almond Butter) (2 balls)
- **Dinner:** Grilled Zucchini and Squash with Avocado Pesto (1 plate)

Key Points for Serving Sizes:

- *Smoothies:* 1 large glass (about 12-16 oz)
- Oatmeal and Porridges: 1 bowl (about 1 cup cooked)
- *Salads and Bowls:* 1 bowl (about 2 cups of mixed ingredients)
- *Wraps:* 1 wrap (using a medium-sized tortilla or wrap)
- *Egg Dishes:* 2 eggs or equivalent protein serving
- *Snacks:* Typically, about 1/4 cup for nuts, seeds, trail mix, or 2 small pieces for energy balls or cookies
- *Dinners:* 1 serving, with a focus on lean proteins (e.g., 1 salmon fillet or 1 chicken breast) and a generous portion of vegetables
- ***This meal plan offers a variety of nutrient-dense, alkaline-forming meals designed to support weight loss while providing ample nutrition and satisfying flavors.***

21-Day Immune-Boosting Meal Plan

Day 1:

- **Breakfast:** Green Goddess Smoothie
- **Lunch:** Kale and Quinoa Salad
- **Dinner:** Roasted Vegetable Medley with Quinoa
- **Snack:** Almond Butter Energy Balls

Day 2:

- **Breakfast:** Chia Seed and Coconut Oatmeal
- **Lunch:** Lentil and Cucumber Salad
- **Dinner:** Grilled Salmon with Roasted Vegetables
- **Snack:** Fruit Salad with Honey-Lemon Dressing

Day 3:

- **Breakfast:** Berry Blast Smoothie
- **Lunch:** Buddha Bowl
- **Dinner:** Lentil and Vegetable Curry
- **Snack:** Alkaline Trail Mix

Day 4:

- **Breakfast:** Spinach and Avocado Oatmeal
- **Lunch:** Avocado and Spinach Salad
- **Dinner:** Tofu Scramble with Spinach and Tomatoes

- **Snack:** Coconut-Almond Energy Bites

Day 5:

- **Breakfast:** Tropical Paradise Smoothie
- **Lunch:** Grilled Vegetable Wrap
- **Dinner:** Chicken Breast with Lemon-Herb Marinade and Steamed Broccoli
- **Snack:** Hummus and Vegetable Sticks

Day 6:

- **Breakfast:** Pumpkin Spice Oatmeal
- **Lunch:** Beetroot and Goat Cheese Salad
- **Dinner:** Shrimp Scampi with Zucchini Noodles
- **Snack:** Cashew Cream Tartlets

Day 7:

- **Breakfast:** Avocado Almond Smoothie
- **Lunch:** Power Bowl
- **Dinner:** Cauliflower Steak with Lemon-Herb Sauce
- **Snack:** Date and Nut Energy Balls

Day 8:

- **Breakfast:** Almond Butter and Berry Oatmeal
- **Lunch:** Spinach and Feta Wrap
- **Dinner:** Roasted Beet Salad with Goat Cheese and Walnuts

- **Snack:** Avocado Dip and Whole Grain Tortilla Chips

Day 9:

- **Breakfast:** Tropical Fruit Oatmeal
- **Lunch:** Hummus and Veggie Wrap
- **Dinner:** Black Bean and Corn Salad with Grilled Chicken
- **Snack:** Lemon Blueberry Sorbet

Day 10:

- **Breakfast:** Spinach and Cucumber Smoothie
- **Lunch:** Lentil Soup
- **Dinner:** Baked Chicken Breast with Roasted Brussels Sprouts
- **Snack:** Chia Seed Raspberry Jam Bars

Day 11:

Breakfast: Oatmeal with Chia Seeds and Coconut Milk

Lunch: Grain Bowl with Avocado and Vegetables

Dinner: Roasted Vegetable Soup with Coconut Milk

Snack: Sweet and Salty Trail Mix

Day 12:

Breakfast: Buckwheat Pancakes with Fruit

Lunch: Avocado and Tomato Wrap

Dinner: Grilled Zucchini and Squash with Avocado Pesto

Snack: Pumpkin Seed Brittle

Day 13:

- **Breakfast:** Green Goddess Smoothie
- **Lunch:** Salad Bowl with Mixed Greens and Quinoa
- **Dinner:** Turkey Burgers with Avocado Mayo and Sweet Potato Fries
- **Snack:** Coconut Almond Flour Cookies

Day 14:

- **Breakfast:** Avocado Toast with Lemon and Herbs
- **Lunch:** Roasted Vegetable Salad
- **Dinner:** Lentil and Vegetable Chili
- **Snack:** Mango Avocado Ice Cream

Day 15:

- **Breakfast:** Chia Seed Pudding with Berries
- **Lunch:** Hummus and Veggie Wrap
- **Dinner:** Beef Stir-Fry with Brown Rice and Vegetables
- **Snack:** Raspberry Lemon Tart

Day 16:

- **Breakfast:** Tropical Paradise Smoothie

- **Lunch:** Lentil and Quinoa Wrap
- **Dinner:** Avocado and Spinach Salad with Grilled Chicken
- **Snack:** Roasted Vegetable Chips

Day 17:

- **Breakfast:** Spinach and Cucumber Smoothie
- **Lunch:** Buddha Bowl with Roasted Vegetables and Quinoa
- **Dinner:** Grilled Salmon with Roasted Asparagus and Lemon-Dill Sauce
- **Snack:** Alkaline Berry Smoothie Bowl

Day 18:

- **Breakfast:** Almond Butter Energy Balls with a Side of Fresh Fruit
- **Lunch:** Power Bowl with Mixed Greens, Avocado, and Chickpeas
- **Dinner:** Tofu Stir-Fry with Spinach and Tomatoes
- **Snack:** Banana Bread with Almond Flour

Day 19:

- **Breakfast:** Pumpkin Spice Oatmeal
- **Lunch:** Tomato Soup with a Side Salad
- **Dinner:** Zucchini Boats Filled with Spinach, Feta, and Tomatoes
- **Snack:** Almond Flour Chocolate Cake

Day 20:

- **Breakfast:** Berry Blast Smoothie
- **Lunch:** Spinach and Feta Wrap
- **Dinner:** Fish Tacos with Avocado Salsa and Lime Crema
- **Snack:** Chia Seed Almond Pudding

Day 21:

- **Breakfast:** Avocado Toast with a Poached Egg
- **Lunch:** Beetroot and Goat Cheese Salad
- **Dinner:** Roasted Vegetable Medley with Quinoa and Lemon-Herb Sauce
- **Snack:** Avocado Chocolate Mousse

This meal plan incorporates a variety of immune-boosting foods rich in vitamins, minerals, and antioxidants while avoiding inflammatory foods. It provides a balanced and nutritious approach to enhancing immune function, maintaining energy levels, and supporting overall health.

21-Day Anti-Inflammatory Meal Plan

Day 1:

- **Breakfast:** Green Goddess Smoothie
- **Lunch:** Kale and Quinoa Salad
- **Snack:** Almond Butter Energy Balls
- **Dinner:** Roasted Vegetable Medley with Quinoa

Day 2:

- **Breakfast:** Chia Seed and Coconut Oatmeal
- **Lunch:** Avocado and Spinach Salad
- **Snack:** Fruit Salad with Honey-Lemon Dressing
- **Dinner:** Grilled Salmon with Roasted Vegetables

Day 3:

- **Breakfast:** Avocado Almond Smoothie
- **Lunch:** Lentil and Cucumber Salad
- **Snack:** Alkaline Trail Mix
- **Dinner:** Lentil and Vegetable Curry

Day 4:

- **Breakfast:** Spinach and Avocado Oatmeal
- **Lunch:** Buddha Bowl
- **Snack:** Date and Nut Energy Balls
- **Dinner:** Stir-Fried Vegetables with Tofu

Day 5:

- **Breakfast:** Tropical Paradise Smoothie
- **Lunch:** Roasted Vegetable Salad
- **Snack:** Hummus and Vegetable Sticks
- **Dinner:** Grilled Zucchini and Squash with Avocado Pesto

Day 6:

- **Breakfast:** Almond Butter and Berry Oatmeal
- **Lunch:** Hummus and Veggie Wrap
- **Snack:** Chia Seed Energy Balls
- **Dinner:** Chicken Breast with Lemon-Herb Marinade and Steamed Broccoli

Day 7:

- **Breakfast:** Berry Blast Smoothie
- **Lunch:** Beetroot and Goat Cheese Salad
- **Snack:** Roasted Vegetable Chips
- **Dinner:** Baked Chicken Breast with Roasted Brussels Sprouts

Day 8:

- **Breakfast:** Oatmeal with Pumpkin Spice
- **Lunch:** Power Bowl
- **Snack:** Cashew Cream Tartlets
- **Dinner:** Cauliflower Steak with Lemon-Herb Sauce

Day 9:

- **Breakfast:** Tropical Fruit Oatmeal
- **Lunch:** Avocado and Tomato Wrap
- **Snack:** Avocado Dip and Whole Grain Tortilla Chips
- **Dinner:** Shrimp Scampi with Zucchini Noodles

Day 10:

- **Breakfast:** Avocado Toast with a Poached Egg
- **Lunch:** Smoothie Bowl
- **Snack:** Sweet and Salty Trail Mix
- **Dinner:** Roasted Beet Salad with Goat Cheese and Walnuts

Day 11:

- **Breakfast:** Chia Seed Pudding with Egg Whites
- **Lunch:** Salad Bowl
- **Snack:** Coconut-Almond Energy Bites
- **Dinner:** Lentil Soup

Day 12:

- **Breakfast:** Green Goddess Smoothie
- **Lunch:** Grain Bowl
- **Snack:** Zucchini Bread with Chia Seeds
- **Dinner:** Salmon with Roasted Asparagus and Lemon-Dill Sauce

Day 13:

- **Breakfast:** Scrambled Eggs with Spinach and Tomatoes
- **Lunch:** Spinach and Feta Wrap
- **Snack:** Almond Butter and Banana Bites
- **Dinner:** Turkey Burgers with Avocado Mayo and Sweet Potato Fries

Day 14:

- **Breakfast:** Oatmeal with Chia Seed and Coconut
- **Lunch:** Avocado and Spinach Salad
- **Snack:** Avocado Spinach Smoothie
- **Dinner:** Fish Tacos with Avocado Salsa and Lime Crema

Day 15:

- **Breakfast:** Berry Blast Smoothie
- **Lunch:** Lentil and Quinoa Wrap
- **Snack:** Chia Seed Almond Pudding
- **Dinner:** Black Bean and Corn Salad with Grilled Chicken

Day 16:

- **Breakfast:** Spinach and Cucumber Smoothie
- **Lunch:** Grilled Vegetable Wrap
- **Snack:** Baked Banana Bread with Almond Flour
- **Dinner:** Grilled Salmon with Roasted Vegetables

Day 17:

- **Breakfast:** Tropical Paradise Smoothie
- **Lunch:** Coconut Curry Soup
- **Snack:** Raspberry Lemon Tart
- **Dinner:** Asparagus and Salmon Salad with Lemon-Dill Dressing

Day 18:

- **Breakfast:** Pumpkin Spice Oatmeal
- **Lunch:** Roasted Vegetable Soup with Coconut Milk
- **Snack:** Alkaline Apple Crisp
- **Dinner:** Lentil and Vegetable Chili

Day 19:

- **Breakfast:** Avocado Toast with Lemon and Herbs
- **Lunch:** Broccoli Cheddar Soup
- **Snack:** Mango Avocado Ice Cream
- **Dinner:** Beef Stir-Fry with Brown Rice and Vegetables

Day 20:

- **Breakfast:** Almond Butter and Berry Oatmeal

- **Lunch:** Hummus and Veggie Wrap
- **Snack:** Lemon Blueberry Sorbet
- **Dinner:** Tofu Scramble with Spinach and Tomatoes

Day 21:

- **Breakfast:** Green Goddess Smoothie
- **Lunch:** Spinach and Feta Salad with Lemon Vinaigrette
- **Snack:** Pumpkin Seed Brittle
- **Dinner:** Cauliflower Pizza with Marinara Sauce and Vegetables

<u>Key Features of the Meal Plan:</u>

- *High in Antioxidants:* The inclusion of a variety of fruits and vegetables ensures a rich supply of antioxidants, which help to fight inflammation.
- *Healthy Fats:* The use of avocados, nuts, seeds, and olive oil provides anti-inflammatory omega-3 fatty acids.
- *Spices and Herbs*: Recipes include anti-inflammatory spices like turmeric, ginger, and garlic, known to reduce inflammation.
- *Whole Grains and Legumes:* Foods like quinoa, lentils, and brown rice are included to provide fiber and maintain low glycemic levels.
- *Low Refined Carbs and Sugars:* The plan minimizes refined carbs and sugars to help reduce inflammation.

By following this 21-day anti-inflammatory meal plan, individuals can reduce inflammation, enhance their overall health, and potentially manage conditions associated with chronic inflammation.

Alkaline Food Chart

Category	Highly Alkaline Foods	Moderately Alkaline Foods	Acidic Foods to Limit/Avoid
Fruits	Lemon, Lime, Avocado, Watermelon, Papaya	Apple, Pear, Peach, Cherry, Grapefruit	Oranges, Pineapple, Bananas, Plums
Vegetables	Spinach, Kale, Broccoli, Cucumber, Celery	Zucchini, Green Beans, Carrots, Cauliflower	Potatoes, Corn, Winter Squash, Olives
Leafy Greens	Swiss Chard, Arugula, Lettuce, Dandelion Greens	Collard Greens, Mustard Greens, Beet Greens	None (most leafy greens are alkaline)
Nuts and Seeds	Almonds, Chia Seeds, Flaxseeds	Pumpkin Seeds, Sunflower Seeds	Peanuts, Cashews, Walnuts
Legumes	Lentils, Green Peas, Green Beans	Chickpeas, Black Beans, Pinto Beans	Soybeans, Kidney Beans, Navy Beans
Grains and Pseudo-Grains	Quinoa, Amaranth, Millet, Buckwheat	Spelt, Kamut, Wild Rice	Wheat, White Rice, Barley, Oats
Herbs and Spices	Basil, Parsley, Cilantro, Ginger, Turmeric	Oregano, Thyme, Rosemary, Sage	Nutmeg, Black Pepper, Mustard Seed
Healthy Fats	Extra Virgin Olive Oil, Coconut Oil, Avocado Oil	Flaxseed Oil, Hemp Oil	Butter, Margarine, Processed Vegetable Oils
Sweeteners	Stevia, Raw Honey, Coconut Sugar	Maple Syrup, Agave Nectar	White Sugar, Brown Sugar, Artificial Sweeteners
Beverages	Herbal Teas (Chamomile,	Green Tea, Fresh Vegetable Juices	Coffee, Black Tea, Soft Drinks, Alcohol

	Dandelion), Alkaline Water		
Dairy Alternatives	Almond Milk, Coconut Milk, Hemp Milk	Oat Milk, Rice Milk	Cow's Milk, Cheese, Yogurt
Animal Protein	(Alkaline diet is primarily plant-based)	None (focus on plant-based sources)	Red Meat, Chicken, Pork, Fish
Other	Sea Vegetables (Kelp, Nori), Wheatgrass	Miso, Tofu (in moderation)	Processed Foods, Preserved Meats, Fast Foods

Standard Conversion Chart for an Alkaline Diet

Basic Volume Conversions

Volume	U.S. Customary	Metric	Imperial
1 teaspoon (tsp)	4.93 milliliters (ml)	1 Imperial teaspoon	
1 tablespoon (tbsp)	3 teaspoons	14.79 milliliters (ml)	1 Imperial tablespoon
1 fluid ounce (fl oz)	2 tablespoons	29.57 milliliters (ml)	0.96 Imperial fluid ounces
1 cup (US)	8 fluid ounces	240 milliliters (ml)	0.83 Imperial cups
1 pint (US)	2 cups	473 milliliters (ml)	0.83 Imperial pints
1 quart (US)	4 cups	946 milliliters (ml)	0.83 Imperial quarts
1 gallon (US)	4 quarts	3.785 liters (L)	0.83 Imperial gallons

Weight Conversions

Weight	U.S. Customary	Metric	Imperial
1 ounce (oz)	28.35 grams (g)	1 Imperial ounce	
1 pound (lb)	16 ounces	0.453 kilograms (kg)	1 Imperial pound
1 gram (g)	0.035 ounces	1 gram	
1 kilogram (kg)	2.204 pounds	1 kilogram	

Temperature Conversions

Temperature	Fahrenheit (°F)	Celsius (°C)
Boiling Point of Water	212°F	100°C
Room Temperature	68°F to 72°F	20°C to 22°C
Freezing Point of Water	32°F	0°C
Oven Temperatures:		
- Very Low	200°F	93°C
- Low	250°F	121°C
- Moderate	350°F	177°C
- High	425°F	218°C
- Very High	500°F	260°C

Common Ingredient Conversions

Ingredient	U.S. Customary	Metric
1 cup flour	120 grams (g)	
1 cup sugar	200 grams (g)	
1 cup brown sugar	220 grams (g)	
1 cup rolled oats	90 grams (g)	
1 cup almonds	143 grams (g)	
1 cup quinoa (uncooked)	170 grams (g)	
1 cup chopped vegetables	150 grams (g)	
1 cup cooked rice	200 grams (g)	
1 medium avocado	150 grams (g)	
1 tablespoon chia seeds	12 grams (g)	
1 tablespoon olive oil	13.5 grams (g)	
1 large egg	50 grams (g)	

Liquid Conversions

Liquid	U.S. Customary	Metric

1 cup water	240 milliliters (ml)	
1 cup almond milk	240 milliliters (ml)	
1 cup coconut milk	240 milliliters (ml)	
1 tablespoon lemon juice	15 milliliters (ml)	
1 tablespoon apple cider vinegar	15 milliliters (ml)	

Herbs and Spices Conversions

Herbs and Spices	U.S. Customary	Metric
1 tablespoon fresh herbs	3 teaspoons chopped	
1 teaspoon dried herbs	1 teaspoon	
1 tablespoon ground spices	6 grams (g)	

Usage Tips:

- **Measuring Dry vs. Wet Ingredients:** For dry ingredients like flour and sugar, use a dry measuring cup and level off with a knife. For liquids, use a liquid measuring cup with a spout.
- **Ingredient Substitutions:** When replacing acidic foods with alkaline options, ensure the measurement conversions match the original ingredient's consistency and volume to maintain recipe integrity.
- **Scaling Recipes:** To double or halve a recipe, apply the conversion chart to adjust ingredient amounts accordingly.

This conversion chart will be a valuable resource in your alkaline diet book, helping readers accurately prepare recipes and maintain the proper nutritional balance.

Standard pH Level Measurement Chart for Foods

Understanding pH Levels:

pH Scale: Ranges from 0 to 14, where:

- 0-6: Acidic
- 7: Neutral
- 8-14: Alkaline (Basic)

Alkaline Foods (pH 7.5 to 9.0+)

Food	pH Level	Category
Spinach	9.0	Leafy Green Vegetables
Kale	8.5	Leafy Green Vegetables
Cucumber	8.5	Vegetables
Broccoli	8.2	Vegetables
Avocado	8.0	Fruits
Asparagus	8.0	Vegetables
Lemon (despite acidic taste)	9.0 (alkaline-forming in the body)	Fruits
Watermelon	9.0	Fruits
Celery	9.5	Vegetables
Chlorella (algae)	9.5	Superfoods
Spirulina (algae)	8.5	Superfoods
Almonds	8.0	Nuts
Bell Peppers	8.0	Vegetables

Neutral to Slightly Alkaline Foods (pH 7.0 to 7.5)

Food	pH Level	Category
Quinoa	7.0	Grains
Green Beans	7.0	Vegetables

Lentils	7.2	Legumes
Tofu	7.2	Soy Products
Sweet Potatoes	7.5	Vegetables
Fresh Herbs (Basil, Parsley)	7.5	Herbs
Grapefruit	7.0	Fruits
Apples	7.0	Fruits

Acidic Foods (pH 0 to 6.5) to Avoid or Limit in an Alkaline Diet

Food	pH Level	Category
Beef	5.5	Meat
Pork	5.5	Meat
Chicken	6.5	Meat
Dairy Products (Cheese, Milk)	4.5 - 6.0	Dairy
Coffee	5.0	Beverages
Alcohol (Beer, Wine)	4.0 - 5.0	Beverages
Refined Sugars	2.5	Sweeteners
Processed Foods	4.0 - 5.0	Various
Wheat (Bread, Pasta)	5.5	Grains
Soda	2.5 - 3.0	Beverages
Corn	6.0	Vegetables (Grains)

Usage Tips for Alkaline Diet:

- **Aim for a Balance:** To promote alkalinity, focus on foods with pH levels above 7.0. A diet with 70-80% alkaline-forming foods and 20-30% acidic foods is commonly recommended.
- **Monitor Your pH Levels:** Consider using pH strips to regularly test saliva or urine to gauge your body's pH levels and adjust your diet accordingly.
- **Hydration is Key:** Drink plenty of alkaline water (pH 8.0-9.0) to help maintain an optimal pH balance.

This pH level measurement chart will guide your readers in making informed food choices to maintain an alkaline diet, which can help improve their overall health and well-being.

CALORIE & MACRO TRACKER

MONTH OF :

DATE	MEAL	FOOD/DRINK	SERV	CARBS	PROTEIN	FAT	CALS

CALORIE & MACRO TRACKER

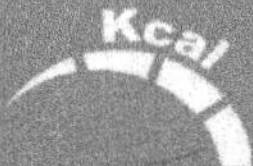
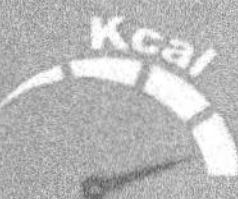

MONTH OF :

DATE	MEAL	FOOD/DRINK	SERV	CARBS	PROTEIN	FAT	CALS

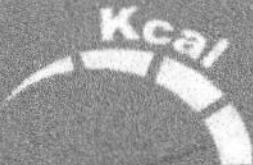
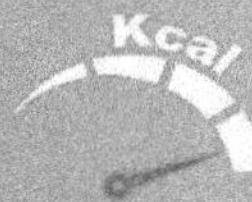

CALORIE & MACRO TRACKER

MONTH OF :

DATE	MEAL	FOOD/DRINK	SERV	CARBS	PROTEIN	FAT	CALS

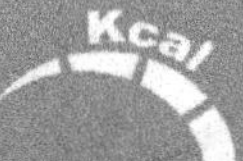
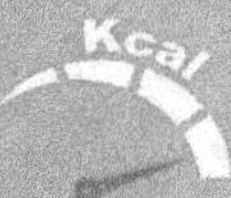

CALORIE & MACRO TRACKER

MONTH OF :

DATE	MEAL	FOOD/DRINK	SERV	CARBS	PROTEIN	FAT	CALS

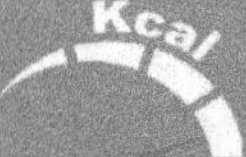

CALORIE & MACRO TRACKER

MONTH OF :

DATE	MEAL	FOOD/DRINK	SERV	CARBS	PROTEIN	FAT	CALS

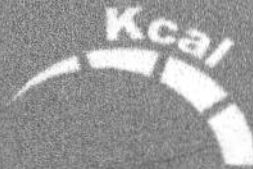
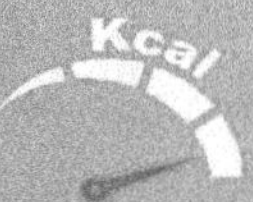

CALORIE & MACRO TRACKER

MONTH OF :

DATE	MEAL	FOOD/DRINK	SERV	CARBS	PROTEIN	FAT	CALS

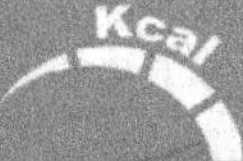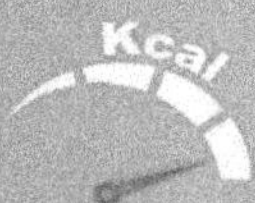

CALORIE & MACRO TRACKER

MONTH OF :

DATE	MEAL	FOOD/DRINK	SERV	CARBS	PROTEIN	FAT	CALS